HOW TO EAT MORE PLANTS

Transform Your Health with
30 Plant-Based Foods per Week
(and Why It's Easier Than You Think)

DR. MEGAN ROSSI

Photographs by Andrew Burton

THE EXPERIMENT

NEW YORK

For Mom: This book is only possible because of you. Thanks for everything.

The Experiment, LLC
220 East 23rd Street, Suite 600
New York, NY 10010-4658
theexperimentpublishing.com

This book contains the opinions and ideas of its authors. It is intended to provide helpful and informative material on the subjects addressed in the book. It is sold with the understanding that the authors and publisher are not engaged in rendering medical, health, or any other kind of personal professional services in the book. The authors and publisher specifically disclaim all responsibility for any liability, loss, or risk—personal or otherwise—that is incurred as a consequence, directly or indirectly, of the use and application of any of the contents of this book.

Names and identifying details have been changed. Any resemblance to actual persons is entirely coincidental.

The Experiment's books are available at special discounts when purchased in bulk for premiums and sales promotions as well as for fund-raising or educational use. For details, contact us at info@theexperimentpublishing.com.

Library of Congress Cataloging-in-Publication Data available upon request

ISBN 978-1-61519-878-8
Ebook ISBN 978-1-61519-879-5

Cover design by Beth Bugler
Cover illustrations by Adobe Stock

Manufactured in China

First printing July 2022
10 9 8 7 6 5 4 3 2 1

Contents

The Diversity Diet: Plant-Based Eating, Redefined

Welcome to a delicious and sustainable way of eating that's good for you, your gut microbes, and the planet. If you're looking for an easy, science-backed way to increase your energy, boost your mood, regulate your digestion, find your happy weight, *and* slash your risk of chronic disease, you're in the right place. As a dietitian and research scientist, I'm here to explain why simply shifting your diet to include more plants could be the best thing you ever do for your health and happiness. And it's an approach based on facts, not fads.

This book will show you how versatile plant-based eating actually is. Forget cutting out or cutting down, I'm going to show you how—and why—*increasing* the number and range of plant foods you eat taps into the very latest scientific discoveries about how your body works best. That's right, eating *more* can improve your health, and my recipes and menu plans will show you just how easy and delicious it really is.

Whether it's something you've been thinking about for a while or a concept you've only just started hearing about, research suggests that more and more of us are interested in exploring plant-based eating. This might mean simply eating more veggie-forward meals each week; cutting down on meat, fish, and other animal-derived products with meatless Mondays; being a "flexitarian" (eating primarily plant-based foods, while still enjoying meat occasionally); or excluding some or all animal products completely, as in vegetarianism or veganism.

According to Google Trends, interest in veganism (an exclusively plant-based diet), increased sevenfold between 2014 and 2019, and it's now getting four times as many searches as vegetarian or gluten-free. The number of vegans in the US quadrupled over this same period, and over the past six years, the number of books related to veganism has increased tenfold.

But we all know that we need to eat more vegetables, and there's lots of information already out there, so what's different about *this* book? Well, first of all, the science. I'm not promoting a fully vegan diet, because research doesn't necessarily support that from a health perspective (more on that in chapter 2). I'm not even suggesting you should go vegetarian, although this book is still for you if you're vegetarian or vegan. What the evidence suggests is that we could all benefit from eating *more* plants, but that doesn't necessarily have to mean *only* plants. So, rather than being about what *not* to eat, this book is all about the many varied and astounding benefits, flavor included, of basing your diet around plants. Because once they're the star attraction, trust me, you'll experience a health transformation.

My first book, *Love Your Gut*, was designed to help people identify and tackle their digestive issues and achieve great gut health. Since it was published, I've received thousands of messages from people whose overall health is flourishing after following the gut health action plan it sets out. Many people also got in touch to ask for a follow-up book that looked more closely at exactly which foods our gut loves and why. So, this book zooms out and speaks to anyone and everyone who simply wants to eat in a way that's more aligned with what our bodies (and gut microbes) need.

And what they definitely need more of is plants.

This book is not about dieting. Nor is it a trendy fad that cuts out food groups or nutrients. Instead, it's your introduction to, and inspiration for, a life-changing way of eating that brings profound, science-backed health benefits in both the short and the long term. Sure, one of those benefits may be weight management, but the benefits linked to nourishing our gut microbes go much further than that—from mood, to skin, to hormones and immunity; they are powerful little things. There's no calorie counting here, no weighing and measuring (of yourself or the foods). In fact, there's none of the cutting out you may see with other eating plans. This approach is enriching, not restricting; inclusive, not exclusive. More plants, more variety, more fiber, more flavor. I call it the Diversity Diet.

In *Love Your Gut*, I wrote about the vital importance of our gut microbiota. Over the past decade, we've made huge leaps in our understanding of what this is and how crucial it is to our overall health. In short, the microbes (including trillions of bacteria, which we cover in more detail on page 14) that live in our gut are key to pretty much all of our body systems, and we need to make sure we have an abundant and diverse range of them to maximize our wellbeing. To do that, we need to nourish them, and what our gut microbes love most of all is an abundant and diverse range of fiber. Where does that come from? You guessed it, plants. Plant-based diversity is more than just a trend—it's based on a ground-breaking scientific discovery, and that's why it's here to stay.

I've created this book as a practical, easy route into plant-based eating, to act as your faithful reference guide as you begin to adopt this approach in your life—whatever that looks like for you. Over the following chapters, I'll take you through what plant-based eating is, what constitutes a "plant food" (prepare to be surprised!) and what the Diversity Diet is all about.

Then, I'll show you all the benefits of choosing this way of eating and highlight the health impact of neglecting the power of plants. I'll give you answers to the common questions and concerns that I hear from my clients, so that you'll have all the information at your disposal—wherever you are on your plant-based journey. This includes my comprehensive "toolkit" of practical evidence-based strategies, from diversity hacks to physical exercises, all of which have successfully transformed the gut health, and overall health, of thousands of people.

Finally, I'll set you on a 28-day plant points challenge, if you choose to accept, and share my recipes and three different menu plans to suit a range of lifestyles. All the dishes are packed with incredible flavors and use readily available ingredients that will not just keep you fuller for longer, but also boost your health and happiness from the inside out.

Now, I realize that some of you will have started your plant-based journey already. You may want to dive straight into the recipes, starting on page 135. Don't let me stop you!

They're all tried-and-tested favorites that will introduce you to some delicious new foods and flavors, without a hefty price tag or the need for chef-level culinary skills. Perhaps you're looking for some added motivation—and love a challenge? If so, you might want to start with the 28-day plant points challenge beginning on page 130. Or you might want to read up on all the background info in the next few chapters and ease yourself into the Diversity Diet more slowly, via my menu plans and gut-loving tips and tricks. Either way, I'm here to help. Whatever your reason for embarking on a plant-based way of eating, and wherever you are on your journey to better health, let's do it together.

I'll be with you every step of the way.

By the end of this book, you'll know . . .

○ **What plant-based eating really means** (hint: it's not plants-only)

○ **Why fiber is the nutrient we all want more of**

○ **Why not all plant-based foods are "healthy"**

○ **Why, when it comes to plants, diversity is key**

○ **How to get your 30 plant points a week,** and then some

○ **How to follow the Diversity Diet** and go easy on your gut

---

○ **How to get going today—** and keep it up for life

○ **Beyond diet:** handy lifestyle tips to nourish your gut microbes

---

○ **Troubleshooting** for those tricky times

○ **More than eighty tasty, plant-based recipes,** for busy people, fueling families, and sensitive guts

Ready? Let's get started.

Part 1: How to Eat More Plants

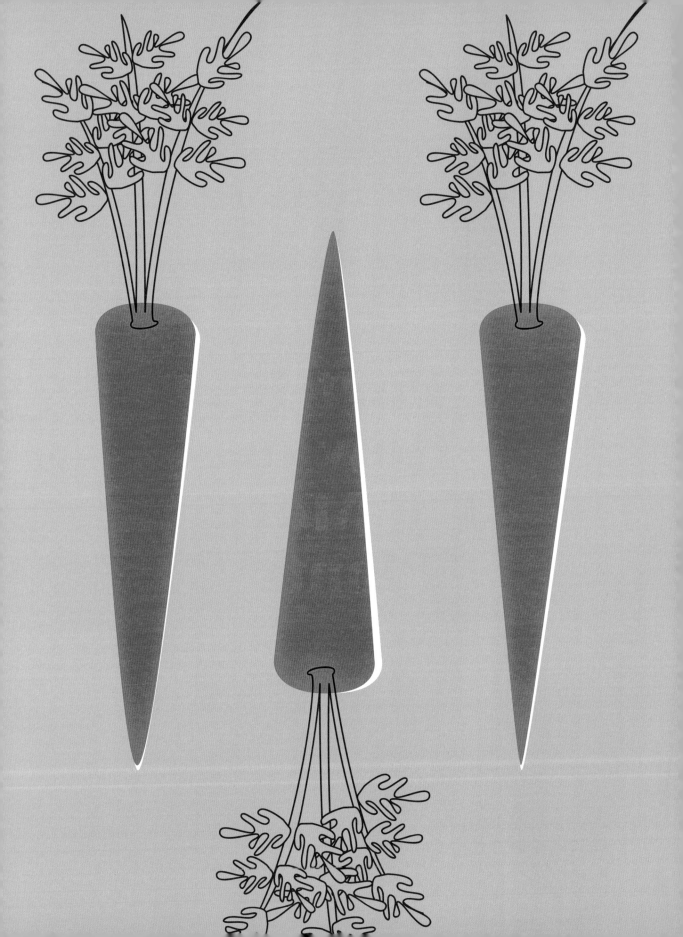

CHAPTER 1

So What *Is* Plant-Based Eating, Exactly?

Is it just me, or are we all constantly bombarded with fad diets, miracle supplements and "superfoods" that fail to live up to their claims? The "next big thing" in health so often turns out to be just another quick fix that doesn't work long-term, and many of us have learned to be skeptical. Good health, we've been made to believe, takes hard work, sacrifice and self-restraint—and there's no such thing as a silver bullet. Except there is, kind of. Because there's one simple way to look after your gut health and reap the cascade of other benefits that it triggers: Eat more plants.

How often do you hear the words "eat" and "more" next to each other when it comes to health advice? That's the beauty of the Diversity Diet as an evidence-based approach—*in*clusion, not *ex*clusion; adding, not cutting out.

Forget What You *Think* It Is

Plant-based eating has become a bit of a hot topic in recent years. But where there's buzz, there's also confusion. What does plant-based eating really mean? Only eating plants? Being vegetarian? Or just eating a bit more green stuff than you did before? And is it a moral choice (*I don't eat animals*)? An environmental one (*I love Mother Earth*)? Or just the latest celeb-backed food trend (*Gwyneth told me to do it*)?

My experience with clients tells me that there can be a lingering prejudice when it comes to going plant-based, whatever you believe that means. For a lot of people, it suggests a holier-than-thou attitude and bland, boring food. Some associate "plant-based" with restriction and missing out on their favorite foods, like birthday cake or grandma's famous biscuits! I'm here to reassure you that none of that applies here. This is not an extreme way of eating; it's quite the opposite, in fact. So let's cut plants some slack, because they really do have so much to offer.

For me, the clue to defining plant-based eating is in the word "based," which means making plant foods the foundation of your diet. In all likelihood, this means eating more of them than you do now. But what you choose to layer on top of that—literally or ideologically—is up to you.

Just Start with Plants

I like to look at plant-based eating as a spectrum. I'm not one for putting labels on the way we eat, and you may not fit within just one "category." To put plant-based eating into context, at one end you have veganism, which avoids all animal produce—meat, seafood, dairy, eggs, honey—and is focused entirely on plant foods. It's totally fine if that's what you want to do and you do it in a healthy, balanced way, which might mean a little extra work (something I touch on later, on page 85). At the other end of the plant-based eating spectrum is flexitarianism, where you eat small amounts of meat—whether that's once a day, once a week, or less frequently—but the greatest proportion of your diet comes from the plant world. Also totally fine.

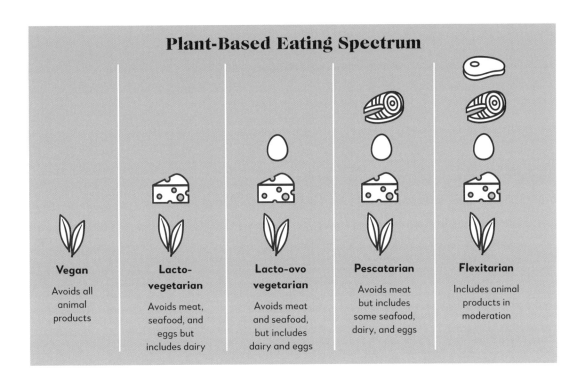

Plant-Based Eating Spectrum

Vegan
Avoids all animal products

Lacto-vegetarian
Avoids meat, seafood, and eggs but includes dairy

Lacto-ovo vegetarian
Avoids meat and seafood, but includes dairy and eggs

Pescatarian
Avoids meat but includes some seafood, dairy, and eggs

Flexitarian
Includes animal products in moderation

In between, there are those who build on their plant foundation with eggs, fermented dairy, fish, and so on. And you can guess what I'm going to say here . . . wherever you sit on the plant-based eating spectrum is absolutely *fine*.

In truth, including some animal foods in your diet can be a valuable way to decrease your risk of nutritional deficiencies. This is evidenced by the "planetary health diet," developed by a board of independent researchers from sixteen countries, as a result of thousands of scientific papers. It establishes a universally healthy reference diet, which takes into account the nutritional needs and overall health of humans and, importantly, considers the environment and long-term sustainability. And guess what, the diet does include some animal foods, albeit in much smaller quantities than many of us eat now. So, I am in no way anti-meat. What I am, emphatically, is pro-plants.

When I say eat *more*, it's not just about quantity; it's also about variety. The more diversity, the better. The beauty of the Diversity Diet is it naturally makes your diet more abundant and diverse. Think "plants" and you might immediately picture leafy greens and salads. But as the next chapter, along with my recipes (starting on page 135), will demonstrate, there's a wealth of flavor and color that comes from plants: whole grains, fruits, vegetables, nuts and seeds, legumes (beans and pulses), even herbs and spices (including tea and coffee).

Meet Your Gut Microbiota

Your gut microbiota, or what I call your GM, is the collective name for your gut microbes: the trillions of microorganisms, including bacteria, viruses, fungi, and parasites, that live along your 30-foot (9 m) digestive tract. And they can't get enough of this plant goodness. Your GM isn't just important for healthy digestion; it also, as research is showing, affects pretty much all aspects of your health, from your immunity to your skin and even your brain function (much more on this later).

Your microbes are foodies by nature. Indeed, they're actually key to *making* many of our most tongue-tinglingly flavorful foods: chocolate, coffee, cheese, olives, soy sauce, wine. They love to sample as many different plant-based ingredients as they can. And you should let them, because the evidence shows that the more diverse your diet, the more diverse and adaptable your GM is likely to be.

Why does this matter? Intuitively, we know diversity is key to all aspects of life. It can apply to a sports team (they need defenders as much as attackers) and to our fitness (we need to work all our muscles, not just a chosen few). Or think about the resilience of rain forests: Every living organism plays its part, and upsetting that delicate ecosystem can have huge consequences.

Your gut microbes are no different. A more diverse input creates a stronger output. Think more skills and a greater support network within you. Call them your superpowers or your inner potential—however you refer to them, they're more powerful than all our human cells combined.

Fueled by Fiber

In my first book, *Love Your Gut*, we established that dietary fiber is essentially the backbone of plant-based foods, and it does way more than just keep you regular. We humans can't break down this type of plant-based carbohydrate during digestion, so it passes all the way into the large intestine (the final 5 feet/1.5 m of our digestive tract), where the bulk of our gut microbes live. Another way to think of it is that fiber is one of your GM's favorite types of nutrients.

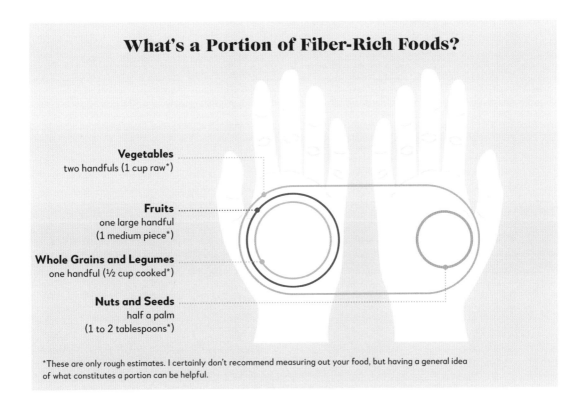

What's a Portion of Fiber-Rich Foods?

Vegetables
two handfuls (1 cup raw*)

Fruits
one large handful
(1 medium piece*)

Whole Grains and Legumes
one handful (½ cup cooked*)

Nuts and Seeds
half a palm
(1 to 2 tablespoons*)

*These are only rough estimates. I certainly don't recommend measuring out your food, but having a general idea of what constitutes a portion can be helpful.

Those microbes are hungry for as many types of fiber as you can feed them. And that's where this book comes in. I'll show you how to pack in more plant fibers than you ever thought possible.

Fiber Facts: Your At-a-Glance Guide to This All-Important Plant Stuff

What is it?

A complex carbohydrate (yes, fiber is a carb!) and the all-important nutrient in plant-based foods. Unlike other carbs, such as starches and sugars, humans can't digest fiber—we simply don't make the right digestive enzymes. That's where our gut microbes come into play: They digest fiber for us.

Where is it found?

Plants! Whole plants. And there are different types of fiber found in different types of plant foods—close to a hundred, in fact—which is why diversity in your food choices is key.

What does it do?

Fiber keeps you regular by bulking out your poop and giving your gut muscles something to work with. It binds to other compounds, lowering cholesterol and preventing blood-sugar spikes. But, perhaps most importantly, it feeds your GM, which breaks down fiber to produce beneficial compounds called short-chain fatty acids (SCFAs). These nourish your gut lining and have been shown to influence immunity, hormones, metabolism, as well as your heart, brain, and more—the list goes on (as you'll learn in chapter 4).

So why all the fuss?

Because chances are you're missing out—and I don't want you to miss all the incredible benefits fiber brings. The recommended daily fiber intake is around 30 grams in most countries. The average intake? Well under 20 grams. Our ancestors, on the other hand, used to clock up about 100 grams a day! Now, I'm not suggesting you have to hit that, but increasing your intake by 50 percent over time is a good place to start.

How do you get 30 grams in a day?

Around three portions of whole grains, two pieces of fruit, five portions of vegetables and one to two portions of nuts, seeds, or legumes per day should do it. If this sounds like a lot, don't worry! You'll automatically get that and more when you follow my easy menu plans (see page 118).

Still need convincing?

Upping your fiber by just 8 grams per day is linked with a reduced risk of heart disease, type 2 diabetes, colon cancer, and death from all causes. Essentially, a well-fed GM really can transform your health.

The Only "Rule" Is Diversity

In this funny old world of social media and hashtags, many of us like to belong to a food tribe. How we choose to eat can become like an identity, a way we introduce ourselves—and something we might fear or feel guilty about deviating from. But that's not necessarily healthy. Healthy is much easier, I promise. We can ditch our quest for perfection and rigid diets, because it really doesn't seem to matter where we sit along the spectrum of plant-based eating.

What does matter is plant-based *diversity*: how many different types of plants you can get in. Forget five a day; we're going to get you into double digits. In fact, my advice is to aim for 30 plant points every week—that's 30 different types of plant foods, which includes whole grains, fruits, vegetables, nuts and seeds, legumes (beans and pulses), and herbs and spices (including tea and coffee).

But don't worry: I promise hitting your diversity goals is easier than you might think.

We'll take it slow and make it fun, easy, and, most importantly, delicious. I've convinced even the most committed meat eaters that adding more plants to their plate is a much tastier way to eat—one of my most satisfying achievements to date!

Rest assured, I'm not going to leave you with just the top-level stuff. In this book, we'll get down to the nitty-gritty and practical aspects. We'll look at what these foods are, how to count your plant points, how the Diversity Diet actually benefits our bodies, how we can make simple changes to our current eating habits, and we'll also resolve any reservations you may have about going plant-based. Whether you're worried about taste, cooking skills, costs, or managing a more sensitive gut, chapter 5 has you covered.

6 Principles of the Diversity Diet

1. **Mostly plants.** Make plants the base of your diet (building on this foundation with eggs, fermented dairy, fish, and more as you like).

2. **Diversity all the way.** Aim for 30+ plant points a week, including whole grains, fruits, vegetables, nuts and seeds, legumes, and herbs and spices.

3. **Go for whole, not refined.** Opt for whole plants that have been minimally processed. More nutrients and less waste: It's a win for you, your microbes, and the planet.

4. **INclusion not EXclusion.** Focus on what you're adding in, not cutting out. It's a science-backed way to transform your relationship with food.

5. **Taste, pause, and enjoy.** If you do, good health and digestion tend to take care of themselves. It's not just about *what* you eat, it's about *how* you eat, too.

6. **Cultivate community.** See each meal as an opportunity to share, connect, and learn. Because eating is about community, culture, and experiences, too.

And that's it! Forget the calorie counting and the inevitable restrictions that the word "diet" typically implies. The Diversity Diet is an easy, delicious, and science-backed way of eating, governed by just six principles. Embrace these and you'll be well on your way to transforming your overall health and happiness.

What 30 plant points actually looks like

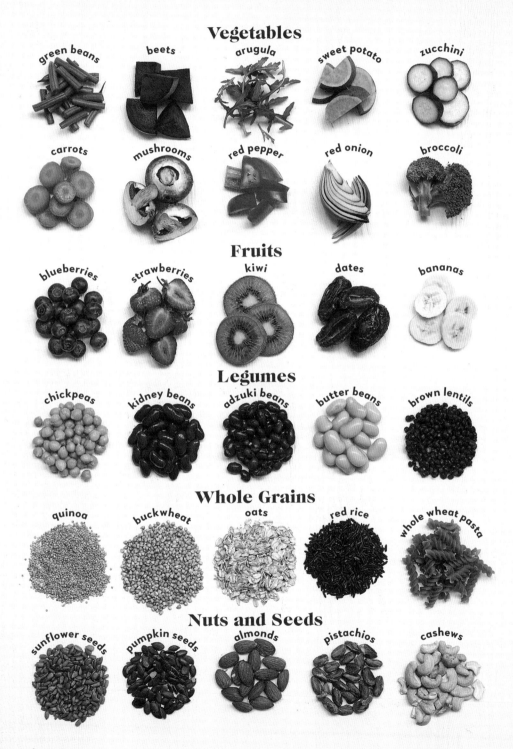

Vegetables

green beans · beets · arugula · sweet potato · zucchini

carrots · mushrooms · red pepper · red onion · broccoli

Fruits

blueberries · strawberries · kiwi · dates · bananas

Legumes

chickpeas · kidney beans · adzuki beans · butter beans · brown lentils

Whole Grains

quinoa · buckwheat · oats · red rice · whole wheat pasta

Nuts and Seeds

sunflower seeds · pumpkin seeds · almonds · pistachios · cashews

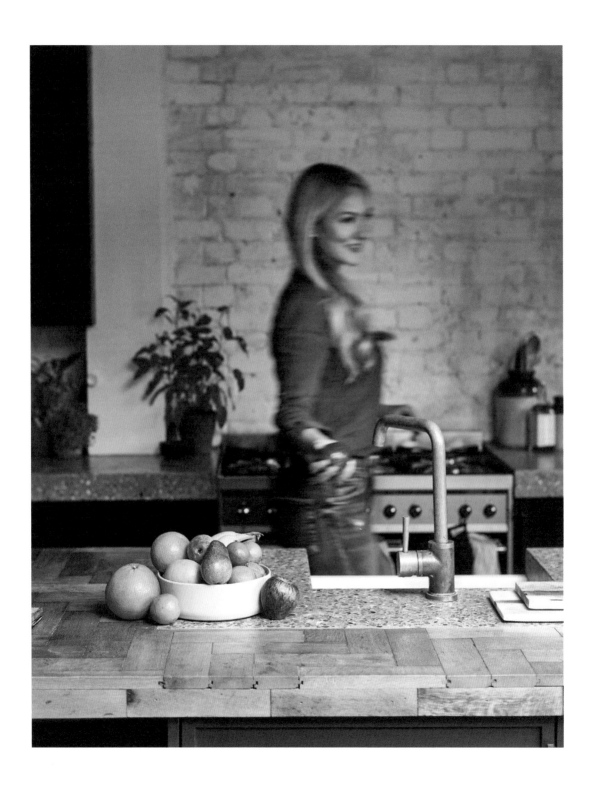

How to Eat More Plants

Learning to Love Plants

So the goal is a diet based mainly on plants. But what if you're just not that into them? Believe me, I've met a lot of people who weren't the biggest plant fans at first. Though eating may seem simple (many of us can down a meal while distracted, without a thought), it can actually be a complex affair. If you were forced to eat boiled Brussels sprouts as a kid, for example, those negative memories may persist into adulthood.

But what if it's purely the taste of certain vegetables that you don't like? There are two things to consider here. First, every food can taste bad if it's not prepped right. There's a world of difference between soggy, overcooked broccoli and lightly steamed, crunchy florets roasted in soy sauce and garlic. Cooking methods matter, especially when it comes to veggies—plus, I'm all about adding the right flavors to plants to make them irresistible. We'll do plenty of this in the recipes in this book.

Second, the way we perceive taste is influenced by a range of factors, from the smell and texture of food to our taste buds, our genes, and perhaps even our microbes. Did you know, for example, that your taste buds adapt and can regenerate every ten or so days? This means a lot of your food preferences are learned, as was the case with David.

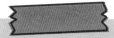

Case Study

I met twenty-nine-year-old David in my clinic, along with his wife, Hannah, who'd made his appointment because they wanted to start trying for a baby. Hannah had read that it wasn't just the woman's diet that could impact fertility; what the man ate mattered, too. David was equally fascinated by it all.

Sitting in front of me was a very drained David, who was a trainee ER doctor coming off a run of night shifts. As we reviewed his diet, David explained that his food choices had gone downhill since he started working in the emergency room, and that he had fallen into the trap of getting post-shift pick-me-ups from the drive-thru of his local fast-food chain. David was all too aware of the benefits of healthy eating, having six months earlier lost his father to a diet-related heart attack at the age of sixty-two. So, for him to improve his diet, it was more about working on behavioral changes.

Together, the three of us came up with a plan that included upping the plant-based protein source in his meal at work (we went with different legumes to increase the satiety factor); having a tasty plant-based snack in his car for his pick-me-up (see my Ultimate Raspberry and White Chocolate Muffins on page 163 and Prebiotic Rocky Road on page 283 for snacks you can make for yourself); and changing his route home to help break the habit of turning in to the drive-thru, where there was not a vegetable in sight.

When I saw David a few weeks later, he told me he'd "relapsed" a few times. But I reassured him that it wasn't all or nothing. If he did stop off for that burger occasionally, there was no need for guilt. Instead, I suggested he implement one simple principle: If he picked up a burger, he had to add two different vegetables to it when he got home.

Five weeks later, a fascinating change had happened. David explained that, after weeks of forgoing the fast food for more wholesome, plant-based meals, he'd decided to treat himself to a super-sized burger one night after a particularly hard shift. It was striking how upset David looked when he recounted that, when he bit into the burger, the taste wasn't as he'd remembered. He didn't get the same kick as before.

By changing his diet, David had allowed his taste buds to change, so the foods he used to crave no longer seemed as delicious. David remarked that the taste change was "like magic"—except it wasn't! It was based on science, and it's something that I see happen time and time again in my clinic.

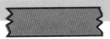

A Matter of Taste

So, how does this work? Well, alongside our taste-bud regeneration, we know that repeated exposure to certain foods is important. Research shows that you can train your taste buds by eating more of the foods you don't (think you) like, particularly for more complex flavors. Think about it: When you were younger, how many times did you take a sip of your parents' coffee or wine, or try an olive or dark chocolate, and think *yuck*? And yet, eventually, you got used to the taste and now might even crave it.

Making these changes gradually is also key. For example, the big cereal companies in the UK have managed to remove over 40 percent of the salt in breakfast cereals since 1998—that's around 240 tons of salt each year! Did their customers object? No, they didn't even notice.

My point is that our food preferences are not set in stone, and our palates can evolve if we let them.

Good for You, Good for the Planet

Finally, let's not forget climate change. While you're feeding your inner ecosystem, you also get the satisfaction of nourishing the global one. Recent research has revealed that a quarter of all global greenhouse gas emissions come from food—and more than half of those come from animal products. What's more, cutting down your meat intake (below 3.5 ounces/100 g per day) reduces your dietary carbon footprint (greenhouse gas emissions) by over 20 percent. So, if you want to go green, tip the balance in favor of plants.

In the next chapter, we'll look at how to do just that.

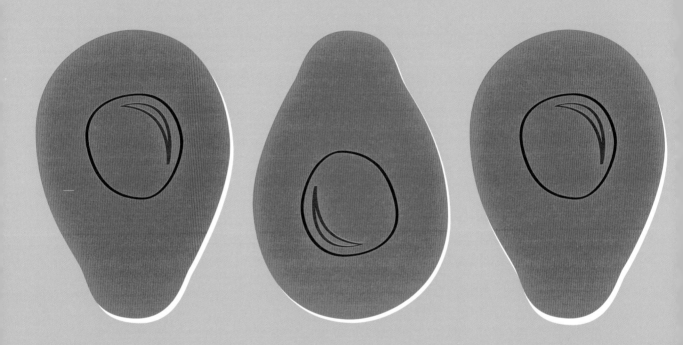

CHAPTER 2

What Are Plant-Based Foods?

Broadly speaking, plant-based foods are any foods that originate from plants. That might sound obvious—well, okay, it *is* obvious— but what I mean is that it's easy just to think of the plants themselves, the leaves. Or even just to think of vegetables and fruit.

But "plant-based" means all parts of a plant and what it produces. I'm talking roots (carrots, ginger), leaves and stems (spinach, arugula, chard), fruit (citrus, berries, apples), whole grains (barley, oats, millet), as well as nuts and seeds (almonds, cashews, sesame, sunflower)—both in their raw forms and everything we can make from them. When you think about plants in this way, a whole new range of produce makes itself available to you. And by proudly proclaiming plant-based foods as the foundation of your diet, you'll feel less like a rabbit and more like a culinary adventurer.

The Super Six

To highlight just how many plant-based foods are out there for your eating pleasure, we can divide them up into six main categories, based on the key nutrients they provide us and our gut microbes.

1. Whole grains
2. Fruits
3. Vegetables
4. Nuts and seeds
5. Legumes
6. Herbs and spices

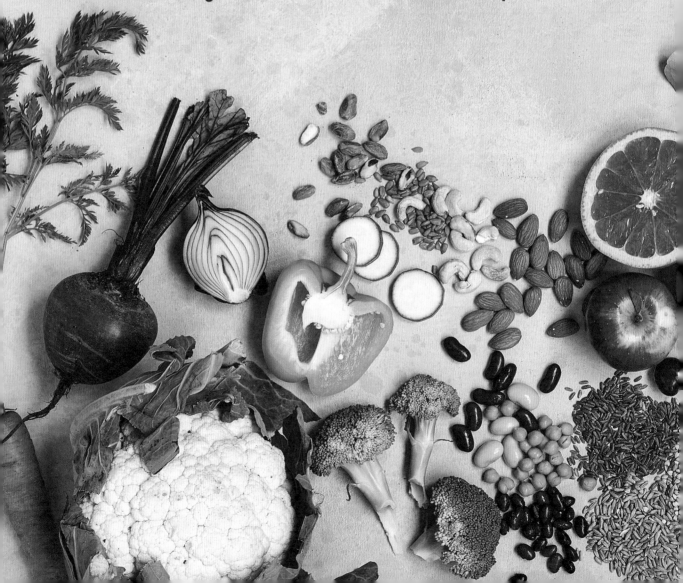

Plant Points: What Counts?

All your Super Six count towards your weekly plant-point goals. Here's a quick guide to adding up your plant points.

| **1 plant food**
=
1 plant point | and | **1 herb or spice**
=
¼ plant point |

- Points are given for each different variety of plant (so if you eat ten strawberries, it only counts as one point).

- Different-colored fruits and vegetables (such as green and red apples or orange, red, and yellow peppers) count different points.

- Fresh, dried, frozen, and canned plant foods (always aim for no added salt and sugar) all count, which makes it even easier for you to get your plant points in.

- Extra virgin olive oil, tea, and coffee count as ¼ point in the same way as herbs and spices do.

- Refined plant foods, such as fruit and vegetable juices, and processed grains don't count because they lack fiber, so try and stick to whole foods, as we'll cover in the following pages.

There's no need to get too caught up on portions at this stage; instead, focus on the diversity. If you eat small amounts of different plant foods throughout the week, chances are they'll add up to a full portion overall.

How many plant points did you get today?

Here's a quick quiz for you. Think back over what you've eaten so far today (or yesterday, if it's still early in the day when you're reading this). How many plant points did you get?

Remember your number, as we'll come back to this at the end of the chapter.

Not All Plants Are Created Equal

As we discussed in the last chapter, plant-based eating is a spectrum, and you don't have to eliminate all or even any animal products to consider your diet plant-based. Keep in mind that it's not necessarily healthier to be vegan or vegetarian. When it comes to your health, the *quality* of the plant-based foods you eat is as important as the quantity.

The Plant-Based Diet Index (PDI)

To put the concept that "plant-based" doesn't automatically equal "healthy" to the test, a team of researchers developed the plant-based diet index (PDI). It's a way of scoring plant foods that essentially classifies them based on the level and nature of processing. The "healthy" PDI (hPDI) positively scores high-quality whole plant foods that have been linked with health benefits. These include minimally processed whole grains, whole fruits, vegetables, nuts and seeds, legumes, and herbs and spices—aka our Super Six. In contrast, the "unhealthy" PDI (uPDI) positively scores low-quality, highly processed plant foods that have been stripped of their whole-food goodness, such as refined grains and cereals, fruit juices, pastries, and concentrated sugars, such as jams and syrups.

The more **high-quality plant foods** eaten, ⬆ **hPDI score**.

The more **low-quality plant foods** eaten, ⬇ **hPDI score**.

The researchers then applied this scoring system to the diets of more than 200,000 people, who were followed for up to twenty-eight years, and what they found was pretty powerful. Those eating healthy plant foods had a lower risk of heart disease (those with the highest hPDI had a 25 percent lower risk than those with the lowest hPDI). In contrast, those eating unhealthy plant foods had an increased risk of heart disease (a 32 percent increased risk in those with the highest uPDI versus the lowest uPDI).

What's more, the hPDI has been linked with gut health—which really isn't that surprising, given that whole plants are loaded with goodness for our microbes, and much of this goodness has been stripped out of the refined alternatives. When it comes to assessing a healthy plant-based diet, then, the level of processing is absolutely key. This underpins the third principle of the Diversity Diet: "Go for whole, not refined."

Hands up if you know someone who's vegetarian or vegan but seems to exist solely on potato chips, cheese pizzas, and highly processed meat substitutes? You may even recognize yourself. Rest assured, you're not alone. Research shows that over 50 percent of the food (in terms of the amount of energy it provides) we eat is ultra-processed. In other words, most of the ingredients are refined parts of whole foods (such as soy protein instead of the whole soybean), combined with additives.

Someone who fit this pattern was twenty-four-year-old Erin:

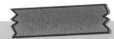

Case study

I met Erin in my clinic, six months after she had decided to go vegan. From both a health and an animal-cruelty perspective, she believed this was the right thing for her. But Erin recounted to me that, four months in, things didn't feel quite right. Not only had she gained 10 pounds (5 kg), but she was also experiencing brain fog and her skin had started to break out more frequently (and not just around her periods like before). She'd also caught two colds that had sent her to bed, despite previously being rather proud of her resilient immune system.

As I reviewed Erin's diet before and after turning vegan, it was clear what had happened. She had fallen into the trap of relying on those convenient animal-food lookalikes—we're talking vegan cheese slices, imitation chicken nuggets, no-beef burgers, and plant-protein shakes. Not only was she having fewer whole plant foods than she'd had previously, she was also overeating ultra-processed vegan alternatives in an attempt to compensate for the flavor of the animal foods she missed.

So what did we do? We switched out a lot of the processed foods for less-processed alternatives. These swaps became really easy once she learned what they were: cashew cheese instead of store-bought vegan cheese (see the Loaded Vegan Nachos on page 233); whole-plant burgers instead of additive-laden soy protein patties (check out the Smoky Beet Burger on page 215), and whole plant-based sources of protein, such as tofu and nuts, instead of refined protein powders ➡

(try the Snickers Smoothie Bowl on page 295). We prioritized nourishing her inner community of gut microbes, while also celebrating the array of flavors that plants have to offer. As for the animal products, I left that up to Erin.

When I reviewed her progress eight weeks later, she explained that she had decided to reintroduce some animal foods, but kept it to just fermented dairy that was sourced from a local farm, as well as small amounts of local and organic meats. Erin also shared her verdict on my beet burgers: "Cheaper, deceivingly quick to make, and they bring a whole other category of flavor to my plate—I'm sold!"

And the health outcome? Erin's weight and skin returned to normal, and she reported: "I feel better—inside and out—than ever before." All from just a few simple tweaks.

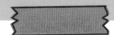

What Do Healthy Plant-Based Foods Provide?

Let's take a look at the beneficial nutrients each plant group offers. The table on page 31 includes the three macronutrients (carbohydrates, proteins, and fats) as well as key essential micronutrients (vitamins and minerals). I've included the main nutrients each group can be considered a good source of, as well as other notable nutrients that contribute to your dietary intake.

It's no secret that you could go into any pharmacy, supermarket, or health food store and buy each micronutrient listed in the table in supplement form. And there is an argument for supporting your diet with certain supplements at certain times in your life, such as if you're pregnant or you're not including all food groups in the case of a vegan diet (see page 85). But here's why popping pills is no substitute for a plant-based diet . . .

There's a wealth of vitamins and minerals contained in each plant food, and these really are team players. They act in synergy with each other—one helping another to be absorbed—and with all the different types of fiber that plant foods contain (remember, fiber is our GM's must-have). This explains why the majority of studies show that micronutrients entering the body through food are generally more beneficial than those in supplement form. The sum of a plant's nutrients is way greater than its parts.

Key Nutrients Found in the Different Plant-Based Food Groups

	Whole grains	Fruits	Vegetables	Nuts and seeds	Legumes
Main distinguishing nutrients	✓ Carbohydrate ✓ Fiber ✓ Manganese ✓ Selenium	✓ Fiber ✓ Vitamin C	✓ Fiber ✓ Folate (B9) ✓ Vitamin A* ✓ Vitamin C ✓ Vitamin K	✓ Fat ✓ Long-chain omega-3 fatty acids ✓ Magnesium ✓ Manganese ✓ Vitamin E	✓ Fiber ✓ Protein ✓ Folate (B9) ✓ Iron ✓ Phosphorus ✓ Thiamine (B1)
Other significant nutrients	✓ Protein ✓ Iron ✓ Magnesium ✓ Niacin (B3) ✓ Phosphorus ✓ Thiamine (B1) ✓ Zinc	✓ Carbohydrate ✓ Folate (B9) ✓ Manganese ✓ Potassium ✓ Vitamin A*	✓ Carbohydrate ✓ Iron ✓ Magnesium ✓ Manganese ✓ Niacin (B3) ✓ Pantothenic acid (B5) ✓ Potassium ✓ Pyridoxine (B6) ✓ Riboflavin (B2)	✓ Fiber ✓ Protein ✓ Iron ✓ Niacin (B3) ✓ Phosphorus ✓ Pyridoxine (B6) ✓ Selenium ✓ Thiamine (B1) ✓ Zinc	✓ Carbohydrate ✓ Magnesium ✓ Manganese ✓ Phosphorus ✓ Pyridoxine (B6) ✓ Selenium ✓ Zinc

*In the form of beta-carotene, which the body converts to vitamin A.

This is just a general guide. Foods within each group vary, and that is the beauty of plant-based diversity.

What about herbs and spices? They don't typically provide us with significant amounts of macro- or micronutrients. But that's no reason to disregard them—they still have plenty to offer! Read on and you'll discover the wonders of phytochemicals . . .

Phytochemicals: A Whole New World of Plant Power

The benefits of plant-based foods go well beyond macro- and micronutrients; plants are full of phytochemicals, too. Phytochemicals are essentially plant chemicals, many of which have been shown to have a host of beneficial effects in the body. There are literally tens of thousands of different phytochemicals, each with different functions. It's these phytochemicals that give plants much of their color, flavor, aroma, and texture. While there's still a lot we don't yet know about phytochemicals, here are five ways that they've been shown to benefit us, with examples of plant sources in bold (based on test-tube studies):

1. Antioxidant and inflammation-quenching powers

These protect our cells against damaging compounds known as free radicals, which can play a role in the aging process and cancer formation, among many other conditions. Phytochemicals with antioxidant activity include allyl sulfides (**onions, leeks, and garlic**), carotenoids (**carrots, tomatoes, and peppers**) and flavonoids (**teas, berries, and kale**).

2. Hormone regulators

Some are hormones themselves, such as melatonin (**black rice, pistachios, and peppers**); others act similarly to hormones, like phytoestrogens (**soy, broccoli, and oranges**); and many interact with hormones, such as indoles and glucosinolates (**cabbages, cauliflower, and Brussels sprouts**), which have been shown to reduce the production of cancer-related hormones.

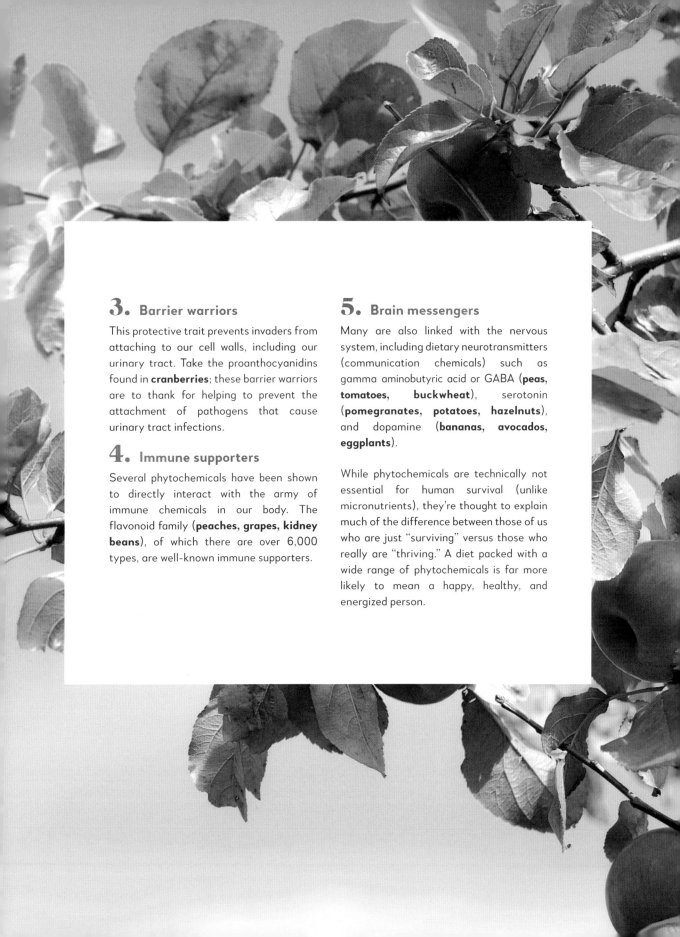

3. Barrier warriors

This protective trait prevents invaders from attaching to our cell walls, including our urinary tract. Take the proanthocyanidins found in **cranberries**; these barrier warriors are to thank for helping to prevent the attachment of pathogens that cause urinary tract infections.

4. Immune supporters

Several phytochemicals have been shown to directly interact with the army of immune chemicals in our body. The flavonoid family (**peaches, grapes, kidney beans**), of which there are over 6,000 types, are well-known immune supporters.

5. Brain messengers

Many are also linked with the nervous system, including dietary neurotransmitters (communication chemicals) such as gamma aminobutyric acid or GABA (**peas, tomatoes, buckwheat**), serotonin (**pomegranates, potatoes, hazelnuts**), and dopamine (**bananas, avocados, eggplants**).

While phytochemicals are technically not essential for human survival (unlike micronutrients), they're thought to explain much of the difference between those of us who are just "surviving" versus those who really are "thriving." A diet packed with a wide range of phytochemicals is far more likely to mean a happy, healthy, and energized person.

And You Thought It Was Just an Apple . . .

They say an apple a day keeps the doctor away and, sure enough, there's a whole pharmacy of amazing ingredients hiding in and under that peel. Let's take a look at how much bang you get for every bite. (And remember, this is just a humble apple—I could provide thousands of examples of plant foods with similarly impressive, yet strikingly different, credentials.)

Yes, apples are a source of carbohydrates, including fiber, vitamins, and minerals, but break it down further and there are around three hundred different phytochemicals packed into that little sphere.

In addition to feeding your gut bacteria with all these fibers and phytochemicals, each apple has also been shown to contain some one hundred million bacteria of its own, too. So eating an apple may very well help make your GM abundant and diverse in more ways than one.

Just as there are lots of varieties of apple—more than 7,500, in fact—there will be variations in the nutrient profile. These days, however, most store-bought apples reflect just a handful of varieties, bred for their sweetness, and most of them contain a smaller amount of phytochemicals compared to older varieties. Additionally, imperfect fruit and vegetables have been shown to contain more phytochemicals. That's because, when a plant faces more stress, it produces more of these great chemicals. What doesn't kill you makes you stronger, right? It's the same for plants! So embrace diversity in your apple choices—show some love to the weird and wonky ones!

An apple is just one example of a plant-based food and all the nutrient diversity to be found within. If you expand this to all the other plant-based foods you eat, filled with countless different phytochemicals, suddenly your diet will look like a magical plant pharmacy!

This is why I'm not a big fan of the term "superfood"—to me, all plants are pretty fantastic.

The Apple Pharmacy

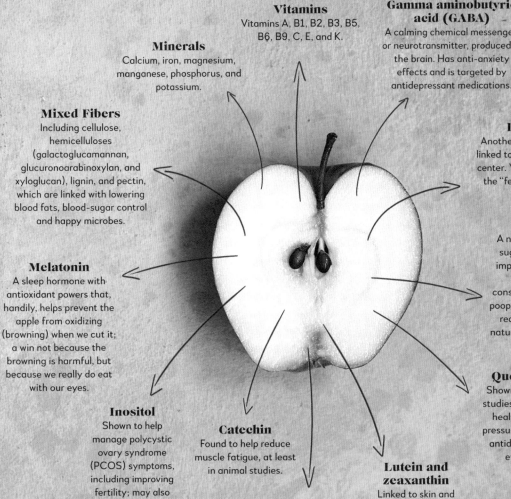

Vitamins
Vitamins A, B1, B2, B3, B5, B6, B9, C, E, and K.

Gamma aminobutyric acid (GABA)
A calming chemical messenger, or neurotransmitter, produced in the brain. Has anti-anxiety effects and is targeted by antidepressant medications.

Minerals
Calcium, iron, magnesium, manganese, phosphorus, and potassium.

Dopamine
Another neurotransmitter, linked to the brain's pleasure center. You might know it as the "feel good" chemical.

Mixed Fibers
Including cellulose, hemicelluloses (galactoglucamannan, glucuronoarabinoxylan, and xyloglucan), lignin, and pectin, which are linked with lowering blood fats, blood-sugar control and happy microbes.

Sorbitol
A natural alternative to sugar that has a lower impact on blood sugars. Also helps with constipation by softening poop (and more commonly recognized as being in nature's laxative, prunes!).

Melatonin
A sleep hormone with antioxidant powers that, handily, helps prevent the apple from oxidizing (browning) when we cut it; a win not because the browning is harmful, but because we really do eat with our eyes.

Quercetin
Shown in animal studies to support healthy blood pressure and have antidepressant effects.

Inositol
Shown to help manage polycystic ovary syndrome (PCOS) symptoms, including improving fertility; may also decrease panic attacks and anxiety.

Catechin
Found to help reduce muscle fatigue, at least in animal studies.

Lutein and zeaxanthin
Linked to skin and eye health.

Chlorogenic acid
Has been linked with weight management by reducing glucose absorption.

Surviving or Thriving?

Recent years have seen a worrying trend surrounding "no need to eat" meal replacements. You know, those drinks marketed at high-flying execs who want all their nutrition without having to stop for meals. Typically, the drinks include all your essential micronutrients, the three macronutrients (carbohydrates, fat, and protein), one of the many types of fibers, as well as an array of additives, such as emulsifiers and sweeteners. To me, they epitomize surviving without thriving, which I found to be the case for thirty-two-year-old Harry:

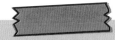

Case Study

Harry was an IT executive. He was the embodiment of "work hard and play hard," but as the years rolled by and the work pressure stacked up, he explained, everything was feeling more difficult. Preparing meals, going to the gym, dating, late nights, early mornings—something had to give. One of his colleagues mentioned these meal-replacement drinks, so he thought he'd give them a go. One fewer thing to worry about.

Three months later, Harry sat in front of me. He couldn't quite understand why, despite the fact that his blood work had come back normal (he was surviving), he felt even worse now, even though he was saving so much time by not cooking, shopping, or chewing. I explained to him that it was likely due to those missing phytochemicals and fibers in his diet. He jumped at the idea of a solution: "Where can I buy them?" And that's when I had to break it to him . . .

The thing about phytochemicals and dietary fibers is that Mother Nature has them hanging over us; we haven't yet figured out how to actually manufacture most of them. To start thriving, Harry was going to have to realize that plant-based foods work in synergy—and he needed to make some time for real food.

Sure enough, after returning to whole food and upping the diversity of plants in his diet, using the hacks on page 94, and managing his stress with the strategies on page 114, he was soon back to his energized self.

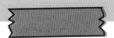

Why Plants = Protein

Protein, one of the three macronutrients, is essential for growing and repairing our body's tissues and making enzymes, hormones, and other chemicals, as well as providing us with some energy. Yet often when we think about protein, we just think of meat.

That's probably because animal products—not just meat, but also fish, eggs, and dairy—are what are called "complete" proteins. This means they contain all nine essential building blocks of protein (aka amino acids) that our bodies can't make on their own. So you could call animal products an easy win, protein-wise. But getting protein from plants really isn't much harder—you just need a range of sources to ensure you get those essential nine.

News flash: Several studies show vegans and vegetarians actually get plenty of protein (recommended to be 0.36 grams per pound/0.8 grams per kilogram of body weight daily). Ignore the outdated stereotype of "hippie" vegans as sandal-wearing weaklings; I've known many a plant-based bodybuilder or endurance athlete, and I imagine you probably do, too.

Sure, if you want to build muscle on a vegan diet, you might have to be a bit clever about the plant sources of protein you consume. But for the vast majority of us non-athletes, just making sure we eat a variety of plant-based foods is all it takes. Yes, a plate of lettuce leaves and cherry tomatoes only contains a couple of grams of protein, but switch that up for a diverse salad such as my Reinvented Couscous Salad (page 210) and you'll be getting around 30 grams of plant-protein per portion, not to mention added flavor.

Ask Google and you'll probably read that rice and beans are the best combo to get the right mix of those essential amino acids. But because you know by now that we're all about diversity, I can assure you that any mix of whole grains and legumes together will help fill the amino acid gaps to deliver a "complete" protein. The more the merrier; variety is key.

Stick to this principle and you won't bore yourself trying to find the perfect combination; it will just come naturally.

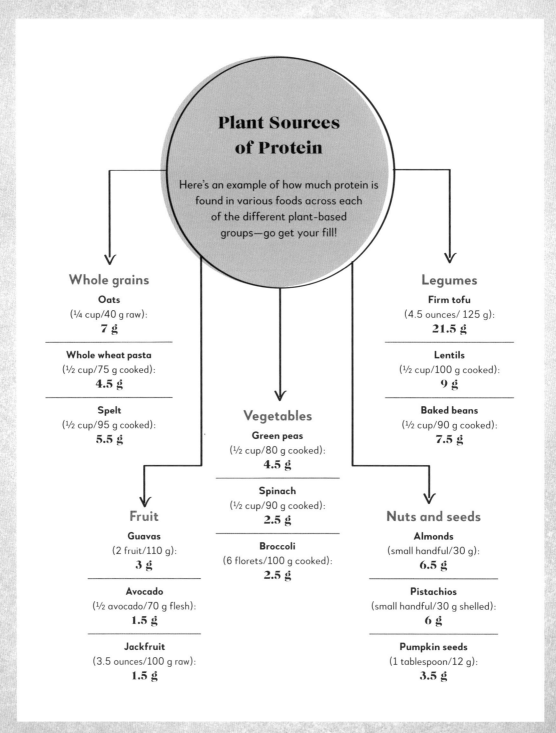

Plant Sources of Protein

Here's an example of how much protein is found in various foods across each of the different plant-based groups—go get your fill!

Whole grains

Oats
(¼ cup/40 g raw):
7 g

Whole wheat pasta
(½ cup/75 g cooked):
4.5 g

Spelt
(½ cup/95 g cooked):
5.5 g

Fruit

Guavas
(2 fruit/110 g):
3 g

Avocado
(½ avocado/70 g flesh):
1.5 g

Jackfruit
(3.5 ounces/100 g raw):
1.5 g

Vegetables

Green peas
(½ cup/80 g cooked):
4.5 g

Spinach
(½ cup/90 g cooked):
2.5 g

Broccoli
(6 florets/100 g cooked):
2.5 g

Legumes

Firm tofu
(4.5 ounces/ 125 g):
21.5 g

Lentils
(½ cup/100 g cooked):
9 g

Baked beans
(½ cup/90 g cooked):
7.5 g

Nuts and seeds

Almonds
(small handful/30 g):
6.5 g

Pistachios
(small handful/30 g shelled):
6 g

Pumpkin seeds
(1 tablespoon/12 g):
3.5 g

Data source: US Department of Agriculture

Remember Those Plant Points?

At the beginning of this chapter I asked you to add up your plant points from across the day. So, how did you score?

I mentioned in chapter 1 that I recommend people aim for thirty—yes, thirty—different plants over the course of a week. So keep counting for seven days and see what your baseline is.

Where does the "thirty a week" come from? It's fueled by research that I've then tested out in my clinic. One of the key studies demonstrated that people who ate at least thirty different plant-based foods a week had more diverse gut microbes than people who ate fewer than ten.

I think it's easy to kid ourselves into thinking we eat a wide variety of foods when really we tend to stick to the same old favorites. Modern life doesn't help—many of us just reorder the same grocery delivery, week in, week out. When was the last time you strolled around a farmers market or even just looked at what the local specialty grocer had in stock? I get that we're creatures of habit and convenience, and I'll admit that I am the same. But our GM needs us to shake it up a bit.

Make your "journey to thirty" fun. The "five-a-day" rule can be a good place to start— but it totally ignores the trillions of microbes living in our gut, which all need different types of plants to flourish. So, stick the plant points planner from page 128 on your fridge and record each new plant point. Go out of your way to find new plant varieties to sample. Kids love challenges like this, and why not get friends, family, or work colleagues involved, too? Check out the 28-day plant points challenge beginning on page 130.

See every meal as an opportunity to add something extra and try something new. There are literally thousands of plants and flavors just waiting for you and your gut microbes to discover them. (Oh, and I say thirty—but once you start on your Diversity Diet journey, don't let me stop you there!)

Gut 101: A Mini Master Class on Your All-Important GM

If you've read my first book, *Love Your Gut*, chances are you've already bonded with your "inner universe" of microbes. But if not, here's a little recap of why these beneficiaries of our plant-based eating are so deserving . . .

First up, we are more microbe than human. Yes, you read that correctly—there are more of them living in us than human cells. There are trillions of microbes that live on and in our bodies—in mini ecosystems in our mouths, reproductive organs, and lungs, and on our skin—but the vast majority are housed in the large intestine, and this is our gut microbiota (GM).

You may have grown up thinking of microbes, such as bacteria, fungi, viruses, and parasites, as enemies to be eliminated, but in truth we need them to survive. Terms like "friendly bacteria" are equally confusing, because really, apart from a small subset of inherently harmful microbes (including SARS-CoV-2, the virus that causes COVID-19), there's no such thing as "good" or "bad" microbes. It's all about how they're balanced.

When it comes to your GM, the technical term for an imbalance of microbes is "dysbiosis." But, because everyone's GM is unique, it's not possible to say exactly what the ultimate balance looks like. What we do know, however, is that when things are out of whack, poor health can result.

Gut Glossary

Microbes

The smallest living organisms we know of; too small to see with the naked eye, so we need a microscope. This explains their scientific name, *micro*organisms. The most common include bacteria, viruses, and fungi. They come in all shapes and sizes, although bacteria are far larger than viruses, around ten to a hundred times.

Microbiota

The community of microbes (you can think of them as the "members" of our inner gut club). One of the most densely populated microbial communities on earth, far exceeding that of soil and the ocean. Together, they weigh around 200 grams.

Metabolome

The handy by-products, such as vitamins and other chemicals, that our microbes produce as they go about their job, including digesting all that fiber. (Using the club analogy, these are the members' voices and belongings.)

Microbiome

The whole environment, including the microbes and the things they produce (not just the members and their things, but the whole club).

What Does Our GM Do for Us?

We know that, generally speaking, the greater the diversity of our GM, the better our overall health and resistance to infection. I always come back to that sports team analogy—you need a breadth of skills to be at the top of your game. And with so many different types of microbes out there (scientists estimate there are tens of thousands of strains of unique bacteria that can dwell in the gut), it's no surprise that we each have a distinct combination within us. Our GM is unique to us, like our fingerprints. Identical twins may share the same human genes, environment, and lifestyle, but their GM will always be different.

As long as it's well supported (that's where this book comes in), our inner universe is a hive of activity, working super-hard at tasks like:

✓ **Munching up fiber** and phytochemicals from the plants we eat.
✓ **Making vitamins** (K and the different Bs), amino acids, hormones, and chemical messengers.
✓ **Training our immune system.**
✓ **Activating and deactivating medicines** and toxins (this explains why, at least in part, people can respond in different ways to the same medications).
✓ **Making chemicals that strengthen** the gut barrier, helping to balance blood sugars, lower blood fats, and regulate appetite.
✓ **Communicating with our brain,** skin, liver, thyroid, heart, and just about every organ in the human body.
✓ **Protecting us against** a proliferation of harmful microbes.
✓ **Assisting gut movement** and function.

In other words, a thriving GM can optimize digestion, immunity, metabolism, hormones, brain function, and gene expression (turning our genes "on and off," affecting what scientists previously thought was our "destiny"). I don't know about you, but since our microbes have this great responsibility, I think we owe it to them to give them as much support as we can.

Whether you think of your GM as your inner universe, Tamagotchi, pet, friend, or simply untapped potential, the next time you sit down to a meal, it's worth acknowledging that you're never just eating for one.

The empowering news is that so much of our GM's health and happiness is in our control. There are many ways we can look after our GM, in terms of what we eat and how we treat it (with things like sleep, stress, and even exercise, which we'll touch on in chapter 6). In fact, our diet and lifestyle choices actually have a much bigger effect on how healthy our GM is than our genetics do. And so far, research indicates that people who consume high-fiber diets, made up of a wide range of whole plant-based foods from the Super Six, typically have the greatest GM diversity and stability. This was the main reason I wrote this book—to spread this landmark discovery beyond the research bubble and help as many people as possible to embrace the far-reaching benefits of the Diversity Diet. And I hope, after reading this book and experiencing it for yourself, you'll feel equally compelled to share it, too.

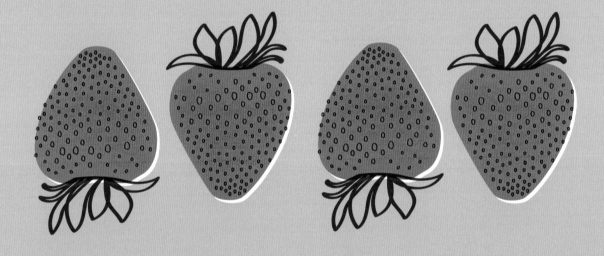

CHAPTER 3

Why Is Going Plant-Based So Important?

My life's work has been devoted to looking at the impact of nutrition on human health, and, let me tell you, what we eat has a *huge* impact—huge! Food is life. So the types of food we eat affect our quality of life. But if you look at our collective health, something's got to give.

All the research I immerse myself in, all the convincing evidence, points to the power of plant-based foods to help us lead healthier lives. This is life-altering stuff, and something we can so easily do to safeguard ourselves against a whole host of lifestyle diseases. Given the relatively simple adjustments involved in making your diet plant-based (remember, this doesn't have to mean cutting out all animal products, and no foods are completely off limits), it's worth taking this seriously. Many of us aren't taking the best care of our health, and yet with a few easy changes—such as by switching half the meat in your pasta sauce for a can of legumes (see page 94 for more switches) or your standard rocky road for my prebiotic version (page 283)—we can.

The Hard-Hitting Facts

We're facing a mental-health crisis—especially in today's world where stress and anxiety are rife. This matters because mental health is one of the main causes of overall disease worldwide; for example, depression is one of the primary drivers of disability. With one in six of us suffering a mental health issue every week, these aren't statistics to be ignored, and thankfully they're something we can change.

The same goes for many other chronic diseases. US diagnoses of diabetes have doubled over the past twenty years. Rates of type 2 diabetes in particular are soaring, along with those for autoimmune diseases and conditions linked to inflammation. These include allergies, rheumatoid arthritis, ulcerative colitis and Crohn's disease, chronic fatigue, fibromyalgia, overactive or underactive thyroid, and many, many more. In fact, six in ten adults in the US have a chronic disease (like heart disease, mental health conditions, and metabolism issues), and four in ten have two or more. Unhealthy diet contributes to approximately 678,000 deaths each year.

Humans are living longer: United Nations records show that, in 1960, the average global life expectancy was fifty-two and a half, and today it's seventy-two. But for many people, these life expectancy gains will be spent mostly burdened with chronic diseases. Where's the fun in extra years if we're not happy or healthy?

The good news is that less than 20 percent of chronic diseases seem to be down to our genetics alone, which means that the other 80 percent are determined by our environment and can be influenced by how we live. In fact, all the conditions we've talked about can be affected, at least in part, by diet. And they have all been linked to GM dysbiosis, which is all too common.

In fact, our GM is linked to most, if not all, of the lifestyle diseases we face today. The more diverse our GM, the greater protection we seem to have from more than seventy chronic conditions. Evidence shows that our GM typically alters with age, exposing us to dysbiosis and the ensuing inflammation that's the root of many of these conditions. But it's not a life sentence. Remember, we can dictate much of our GM diversity by how we treat it, and therefore we have the power to stave off much of this "inflammaging."

The human microbiome is considered the biggest emerging area of research in medical and nutritional science of the past century. A major discovery is happening right before our eyes and revolutionizing our health. Although we don't know the exact nature of all the links to various diseases, and there is still more research to be done, what I can say for sure is that improving our gut health has been shown to improve our general health and happiness in enough studies to have the scientific world convinced that targeting our GM is a game changer for our health. And, according to the scientific evidence, fiber-filled plant-based diversity is the way to fuel just that.

What Are We Eating?

With all the advancements in technology over the last fifty years, it has become cheaper and easier to eat processed foods instead of feeding our gut microbes with the vast array of plants they—and we—need to thrive. While an estimated 300,000 edible plant species are available to humans, more than half of our global energy needs are met by just four: rice, potatoes, wheat, and corn. Many of us have become accustomed to thinking that sticking to these four types each day is "normal," yet the science, the surging rates of chronic diseases, and the way our ancestors ate are certainly telling us a different story.

What we need is to grow a more diverse range of microbes within us to achieve our optimal gut health and reduce our risk of so many of these lifestyle diseases. And how we do that is by reaching beyond just those four plants, to the thousands of other plant-based foods on offer.

5 Reasons to Get Diversifying

1. **A lower risk of nutritional deficiencies:** In the last chapter, I talked about all the micronutrients and phytochemicals in plants. The greater variety you eat, the lower your chance of becoming deficient. Each food provides different essential nutrients. Skip one and you miss out.

2. **Greater pleasure in food:** A more varied diet not only introduces a whole host of nutrients to your plate, it brings amazing tastes to your palate, too. We'll get creative with the Diversity Diet in chapter 6, so you'll soon be enjoying a richness of aromas, flavors, and textures. Why does this matter? Because enjoying our food is linked to better mental health, plus studies demonstrate it also has a positive impact on digestion.

3. **Better overall nutrition:** Many nutrients found in plant foods work together to have an additive benefit. There are so many great examples of how consuming one nutrient helps your absorption of another (see page 49). A limited diet misses out on so much of this teamwork.

4. **A more diverse GM:** It's not just better nutrition for you, but your gut microbes, too. The research shows that the more diverse the nutrients you give your microbes (from the plants you eat—think fibers, prebiotics, and phytochemicals), the more diverse your GM becomes, creating a greater support network within you.

5. **A longer life:** Eating a wide variety of plants doesn't just help us avoid illness—it can actually keep us alive for longer according to research. In fact, one study showed that you can lengthen your life—by as much as a decade!—by eating a diverse plant-based diet. Diversity is key, but researchers saw the best results came from eating more legumes (such as lentils, chickpeas, and kidney beans), more whole grains (such as oats and wild rice), and more nuts (such as pecans and walnuts), because most people weren't eating any of these to start with. The best way to unlock your longevity is, simply put, hiding in a can of chickpeas!

Food Pairings That Enhance Nutrition

For sun protection

Fat increases the absorption of lycopene, a plant chemical with antioxidant powers that can help protect us against sun damage (but don't skip that SPF!). You could eat one lycopene-rich tomato or you could slice it up and have it with some gut-loving extra virgin olive oil or avocado—easily and naturally upping the amount of lycopene available for your skin to take on board.

For more iron

It can be harder to get enough iron if you don't eat meat. Unless you happen to know that vitamin C increases the amount of non-heme iron (found in plant foods) you absorb. It's as easy as adding some vitamin C—rich peppers to that lentil dish, dipping pepper crudités in hummus, or squeezing lemon juice over a salad of dark leafy greens (see my Zucchini and Hazelnut Salad on page 186).

To reduce inflammation

If you like cooking with turmeric, be sure to add a few turns of the pepper mill, too. Curcumin, the active ingredient in turmeric, has been shown to have an anti-inflammatory effect in humans in high doses. In the presence of piperine, a compund found in black pepper, our body's ability to absorb curcumin increases by 2,000 percent! (See my Spicy Red Lentil Bowl on page 242.)

For strong bones

Sun-drenched mushrooms (yes, they're a thing—and high in vitamin D as a result) go nicely with some calcium-set tofu. Or have some salmon (an oily fish and another good source of vitamin D) with spring greens (try the Orange-Glazed Roasted Salmon on page 228). Each will boost your vitamin D intake. And being D-sufficient has been shown to increase your absorption of calcium by around 50 percent. They're both key for a healthy skeleton.

To max out on magnesium

Prebiotic foods—rich in the types of fiber that feed your GM, such as inulin—are known to boost your magnesium absorption. Take advantage by combining seeds and dates (try the Stuffed Dates, Four Ways on page 167) or nuts with artichoke (like in the Creamy Dairy-Free Linguine on page 227).

To build muscle

Get your complete set of protein building blocks (aka amino acids) by combining whole grains with legumes or legumes with nuts or seeds. Try freekeh and mixed beans (see the Mediterranean Hug Soup on page 223) or black beans with cashew cheese (check out the Loaded Vegan Nachos on page 233).

Restrictive Diets = Sensitive Stomachs

Food sensitivities are at an all-time high. If you don't have a food intolerance yourself, I'll bet you know plenty of people who do. But here's the thing: food intolerances or sensitivities are often exacerbated by and even triggered by dietary restrictions.

You know the saying "You are what you eat"? That's never truer than with your GM. Your microbes adapt according to the foods you eat. For example, if your diet is high in meat and processed foods and low in whole plant foods, you'll likely develop a GM profile that is linked not only with diseases such as bowel cancer but also a reduced ability to digest plants. That's because it's not our human cells that digest fiber, it's our microbes, as we touched on in chapter 1. When diverse, our GM is able to produce hundreds of enzymes that break down the many different types of fibers and plant chemicals found in our plant foods. But if your diet is restricted, only a minority group of microbes will thrive, and in turn dominate the community, while other skilful bacteria will be left to starve and eventually die out, narrowing the range of microbes you have.

Diversity breeds diversity. So all these restrictive diets often touted as the key to health and weight loss—paleo, low carb, *no* carb—can be detrimental in the long term. If we starve our GM, when we then eat a bowl of plants, we lack many of the microbes (and therefore their enzymes) needed to digest the different fibers efficiently. This inefficient digestion can, in turn, trigger gut symptoms such as bloating, excess gas, and altered poops.

Now, I'm not saying go out and gorge on the foods that trigger gut symptoms for you—far from it. But keep in mind that no plant food (unless you have a properly diagnosed allergy or celiac disease) should be off the menu long-term.

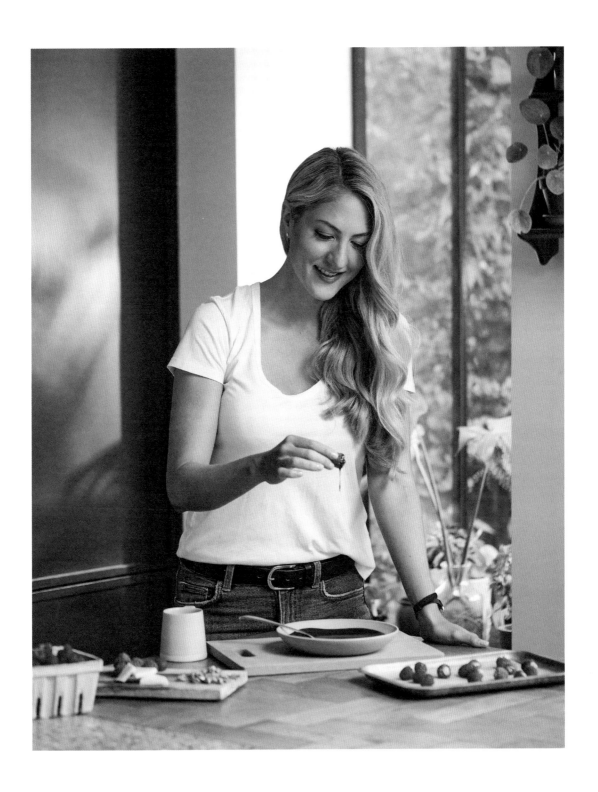

The magic of our gut microbes is that you can generally increase tolerance to plant foods you feel sensitive to. The key is to introduce them gradually and slowly, broadening your exposure and teaching your gut microbes to digest them. And, in turn, this will help to repopulate your GM and increase its diversity. It's like how we build our immunity by coming into contact with germs in smaller doses, rather than living in a bubble.

If you are advised by a dietitian to follow an elimination diet to find the foods you feel intolerant to, the goal should typically be to reintroduce these foods gradually, not permanent elimination. (This is something people—doctors included—often get wrong when it comes to irritable bowel syndrome/IBS and the low-FODMAP diet, and people can end up getting stuck following the restriction stage of the diet for years. Instead, the low-FODMAP diet should include a three-stage approach: restriction, reintroduction, and personalization. For more about the low-FODMAP diet, check out page 126.)

More and more of us are experiencing gut health issues and sensitivities every year. But please don't suffer in silence. Get the help you deserve. For more information and evidence-based strategies, take a look at my website or read my first book, *Love Your Gut*. And if you know that you're sensitive to certain foods—don't worry, plant-based eating is possible for you, too. I've designed the Sensitive Guts menu plan on page 124 to help ease your way into eating more plants at a pace that works for you.

Plants as Medicine

Did you know around a quarter of drugs prescribed worldwide are plant-derived? Just another reason not to underestimate the power of plants. They include aspirin (from willow bark), opiates such as morphine and codeine (from poppies), the heart medication digoxin (from foxgloves), and the antimalarial quinine (from the bark of cinchona trees).

Now, I wouldn't go as far as saying food is medicine—that would be doing both a disservice, as they're very different. Modern medicine can be life-saving, and I certainly wouldn't advise people to just replace their prescribed medication with plants. That said, plant power is real, and nourishing our bodies with plenty of plant goodness can have a profound impact on our health, helping to manage conditions and prevent disease.

A Final Thought

Sure, our health has seen better days. But the good news is we know more now about *why* and *what* we can do about it than at any other time in human history. The typical American diet is simply not good enough. The range of foods we eat is too narrow, our choices are too processed—and this combination is limiting our health potential. But there's a solution: Whole. Diverse. Plants.

We have science on our side, so let's exploit what we know about our GM and do our best to optimize it.

Tip
Some of our microbiome is passed on just as our genes are. By eating more plants now, you won't just be positively affecting your own health—you'll be paying it forward to future generations.

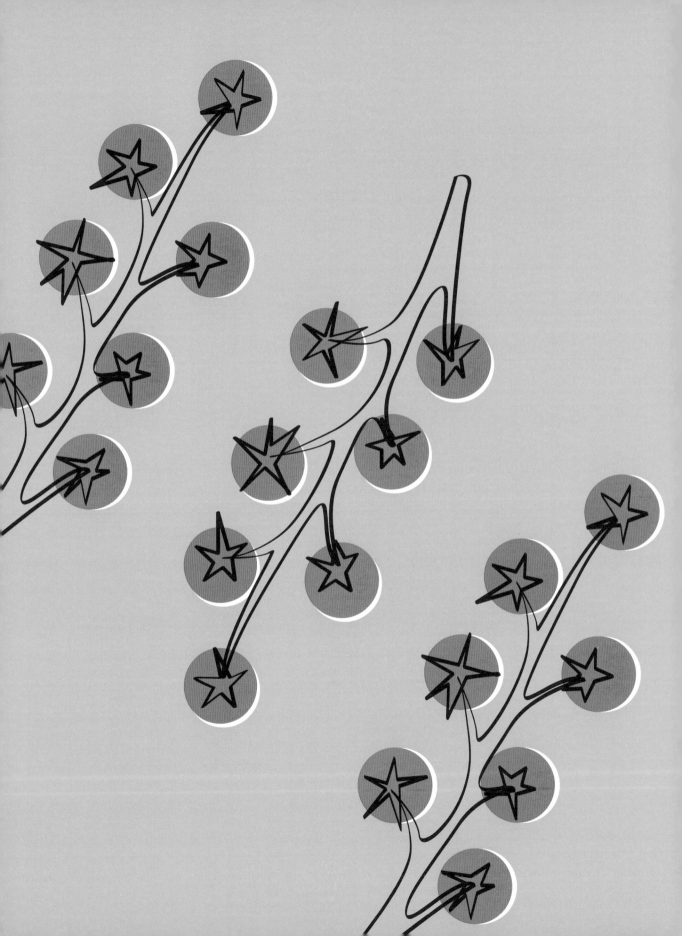

CHAPTER 4

The Plant-Based Benefits

Now we know what the Diversity Diet is, what counts as a healthy plant-based food, and the downside of not adding more plants into your diet. But hey, we're human—which means any change from our norm requires a little extra motivation. And I'm here to give you just that. It's time to ignite your diversity drive by reviewing all the benefits you're likely to experience by embracing those extra plants.

The beauty of focusing on plant-based diversity is that you'll feel benefits immediately, and I've created the recipes in this book to give you all the inspiration and ideas you need to get started. New foods, flavors, textures, colors—I'm talking instant gratification. By eating in this way, you'll start to notice short-term health benefits: better digestion, more energy, less bloating, and more. Before long, the further gains will start to reveal themselves. What's that, you're sleeping better? Your skin's looking good? Fewer aches, pains and seasonal bugs; hormones less haywire? That'll be your well-fed GM returning its thanks! Believe me, I've seen it enough times in clients who've started out skeptical but have increased their plant-based foods and reaped these rewards.

Whatever your current health goals—reducing stress at work, calming tummy troubles, getting to a healthy weight, feeling stronger or more energized, boosting your libido, you name it—the Diversity Diet is likely to help by nourishing your all-important GM.

Once you understand the power and potential of the gut and how it influences—or even controls—so many systems in our body, I think you'll be on board with its diet and lifestyle preferences. To get there, it helps to think of your GM as a great communicator. It has three distinct ways of speaking to your other organs: via the immune system, the nervous system, and the blood and lymph circulation (that helps get rid of waste and toxins). Let's take a look at some of the pathways that get the most traffic, and you'll start to see just how far-reaching those plant-based benefits can be.

➡ **The gut–brain axis**

———————————————————————

➡ **The gut–skin axis**

———————————————————————

➡ **The gut–immune axis**

———————————————————————

➡ **The gut–hormone axis**

———————————————————————

➡ **The gut–metabolism axis**

The Gut-Brain Axis

It's not so hard to imagine a connection between the gut and brain—our digestion and our mental state—if we consider just how many phrases in the English language already exist to describe it. Ever had "butterflies in your stomach" when nervous? Used your "gut instinct" to make a difficult decision? Or felt something so deeply it was "gut-wrenching?"

We've known for over a century that the gut and brain are connected—not just metaphorically, but also literally, thanks to the impressive web of hundreds of millions of nerves that connect the two, known as the enteric nervous system (ENS). In fact, it's the ENS that originally earned the gut its title as our "second brain," because, unlike other organs in the body, the ENS can control the gut independently from our "primary" brain (aka the central nervous system or CNS). But it's only been in more recent years that science has uncovered a new key player, and perhaps even the controller, of this intimate relationship: our gut microbiome. And this has become an understandably hot topic.

While research into the role of our GM is still at the new, exciting, and so-much-still-to-learn stage, there's enough evidence from studies conducted on humans to recommend eating more plants to reduce the risk of, and even help treat, mental health and neurological conditions. Disruption along the gut–brain axis has, for example, been associated with disorders including stress, depression and anxiety, irritable bowel syndrome (IBS), autism, schizophrenia, and Parkinson's and Alzheimer's diseases. There's even evidence that the state of your GM could be used to predict your risk of depression, how long your symptoms last, and how well you recover.

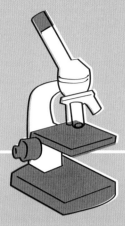

Study Snippet

I couldn't talk about the gut–brain axis without sharing one of my favorite scientific studies. If you're not already acquainted, let me introduce you to the "SMILES" trial — a landmark study investigating whether changing our diets in favor of whole plants could help manage depression. Here is what you need to know:

What they did

People with moderate to severe depression were randomized to receive either psychotherapy (the control group) or a Mediterranean diet full of plant-based diversity for twelve weeks. All of the patients continued to take their antidepressant medication throughout the study.

The results

Those in the diet group were four times more likely to be in remission (based on clinical questionnaires) after twelve weeks. This highlights that diet is best used along with medication as an additional or early-stage therapy. Further studies have since reaffirmed this finding—that upping your plants and diversity can have a positive impact on mental health.

Key takeaway

Those following the diet full of plant-based foods, including all of the Super Six plant food groups (alongside lean meats, fish, eggs, and fermented dairy)—which provided three times more fiber than many of us eat regularly—saw a significant improvement in their mental health. This supports what I regularly see in my clinic: Whether you have depression or you'd just like to safeguard your emotional state, shifting your diet in favor of whole plants can really help.

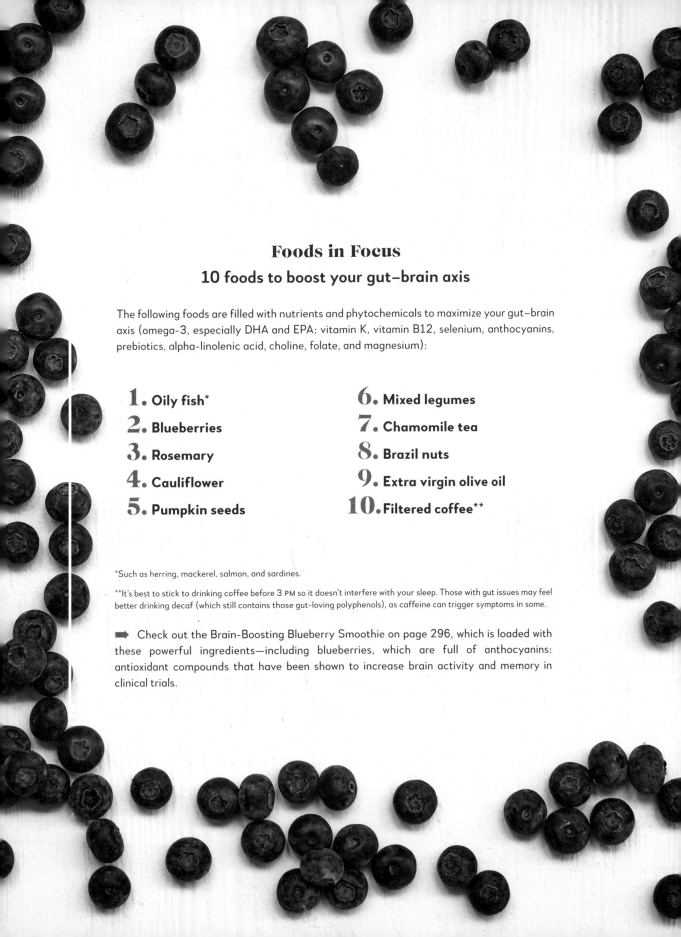

Foods in Focus
10 foods to boost your gut–brain axis

The following foods are filled with nutrients and phytochemicals to maximize your gut–brain axis (omega-3, especially DHA and EPA; vitamin K, vitamin B12, selenium, anthocyanins, prebiotics, alpha-linolenic acid, choline, folate, and magnesium):

1. Oily fish*
2. Blueberries
3. Rosemary
4. Cauliflower
5. Pumpkin seeds
6. Mixed legumes
7. Chamomile tea
8. Brazil nuts
9. Extra virgin olive oil
10. Filtered coffee**

*Such as herring, mackerel, salmon, and sardines.

**It's best to stick to drinking coffee before 3 PM so it doesn't interfere with your sleep. Those with gut issues may feel better drinking decaf (which still contains those gut-loving polyphenols), as caffeine can trigger symptoms in some.

➡ Check out the Brain-Boosting Blueberry Smoothie on page 296, which is loaded with these powerful ingredients—including blueberries, which are full of anthocyanins: antioxidant compounds that have been shown to increase brain activity and memory in clinical trials.

The Gut–Skin Axis

There's a two-way conversation going on between our microbes and our skin (just like with the brain). And when you think about it, the gut and skin have a lot in common: They're both key players in defending the rest of our body from pathogenic invaders; they house a diverse community of microbes; and they're also in a constant state of renewal, with parts of their linings shedding roughly every week and month, respectively, making them very hungry for nutrition.

What we eat and how we treat our GM often plays out on our skin—as you may have witnessed after a few days of not eating many plant-based foods or having one too many glasses of wine. After all, our skin is an organ that relies on what we feed it to stay alive. One of the earliest observations of this dependency was with scurvy: A doctor in the eighteenth century discovered that citrus fruit (rich in vitamin C) could cure sailors of this disease, one of the first signs of which was skin rashes and bruise-like spots.

Similarly, for skin conditions such as acne, there is a growing body of evidence suggesting that not enough "healthy" plant-based foods, too many "unhealthy" plant-based foods like fruit juice and white bread, and large amounts of non-fermented dairy (particularly, it seems, skim milk) may exacerbate acne through alterations in hormones, among other pathways. That being said, there's no evidence that food alone causes acne, nor that enjoying these foods in moderation as part of your Diversity Diet will make acne worse. In fact, the stress of aiming for diet "perfection" in itself can be enough to make your skin break out, thanks to the pesky stress hormone cortisol.

Most of our gut–skin communication happens via the immune system. Simply put, an unbalanced GM (dysbiosis) is thought to set off a response from the immune system, triggering inflammation, which is normally there to protect us from injury or illness. But, like the stress response, inflammation becomes a problem when it's triggered too often and left switched on at a low level over time. Many skin conditions—eczema, rosacea, acne, psoriasis, dermatitis, even premature aging—are inflammatory in origin, so it figures that a limited GM, lacking in diversity, could be involved.

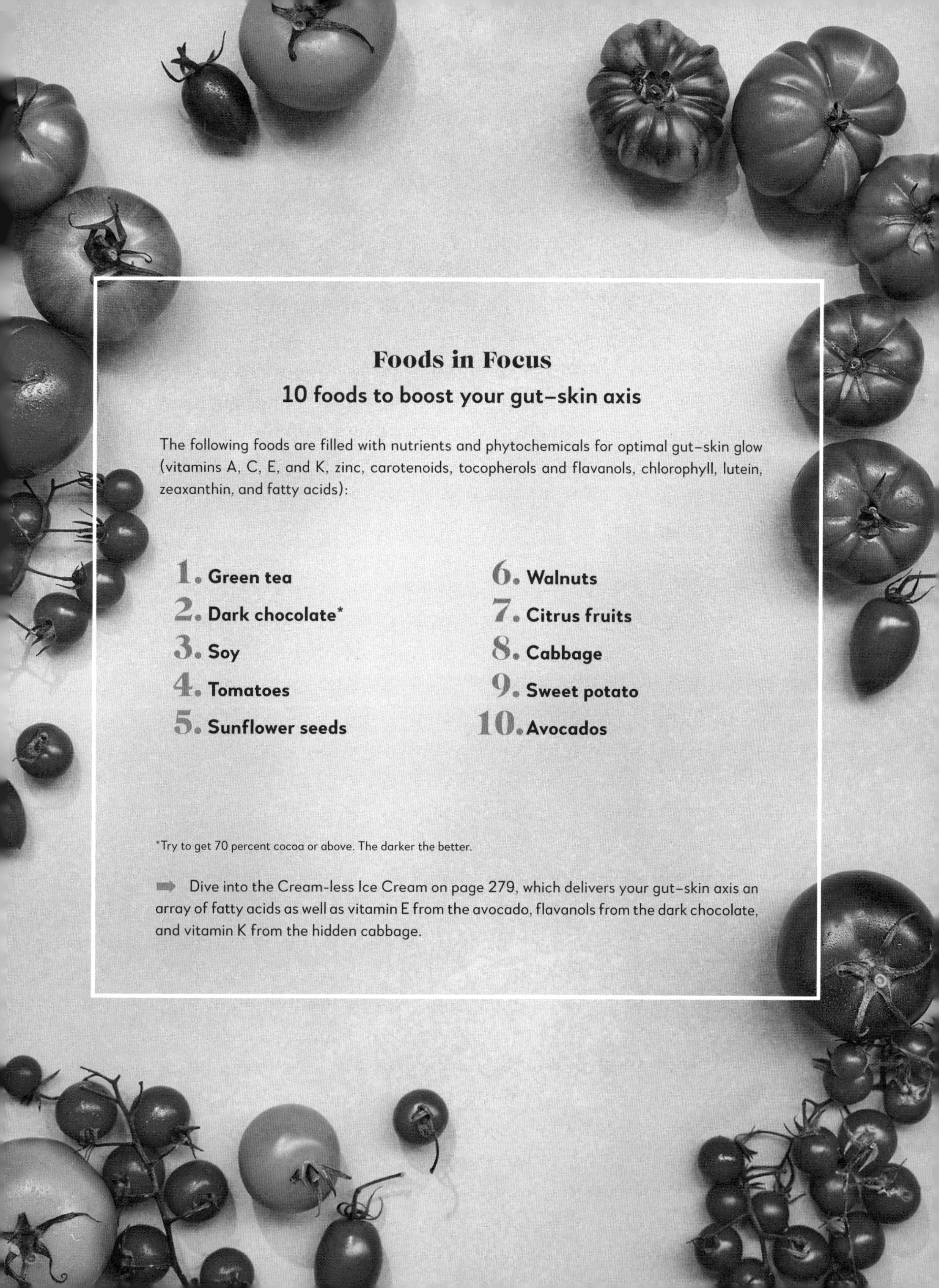

Foods in Focus
10 foods to boost your gut–skin axis

The following foods are filled with nutrients and phytochemicals for optimal gut–skin glow (vitamins A, C, E, and K, zinc, carotenoids, tocopherols and flavanols, chlorophyll, lutein, zeaxanthin, and fatty acids):

1. Green tea
2. Dark chocolate*
3. Soy
4. Tomatoes
5. Sunflower seeds

6. Walnuts
7. Citrus fruits
8. Cabbage
9. Sweet potato
10. Avocados

*Try to get 70 percent cocoa or above. The darker the better.

➡ Dive into the Cream-less Ice Cream on page 279, which delivers your gut–skin axis an array of fatty acids as well as vitamin E from the avocado, flavanols from the dark chocolate, and vitamin K from the hidden cabbage.

If we have a more diverse GM, our microbes keep each other in line and instead can have anti-inflammatory effects. This is partly thanks to the short-chain fatty acids (SCFA) released when they digest fiber (as explained on page 16), which are thought to help our skin counteract some of the environmental damage it faces.

Skin Aging

Even if you don't have any specific skin concerns, it's worth knowing that the gut–skin axis is involved in something we'd all rather slow down: skin aging. Polyphenols—the beneficial plant chemicals that mostly rely on our GM for absorption in the body (and therefore into the skin)—have also been shown to improve the appearance of aging. One study using polyphenols from cocoa (hello, dark chocolate!) showed reduced facial wrinkles and improved elasticity after twenty-four weeks, compared to placebo (non-polyphenol intervention).

Another study suggested that our skin microbiota can even predict our age, and another found that eating more plants was linked with improved telomere length, a marker of aging. Now, Botox or that extra portion of vegetables? I'll let you decide . . .

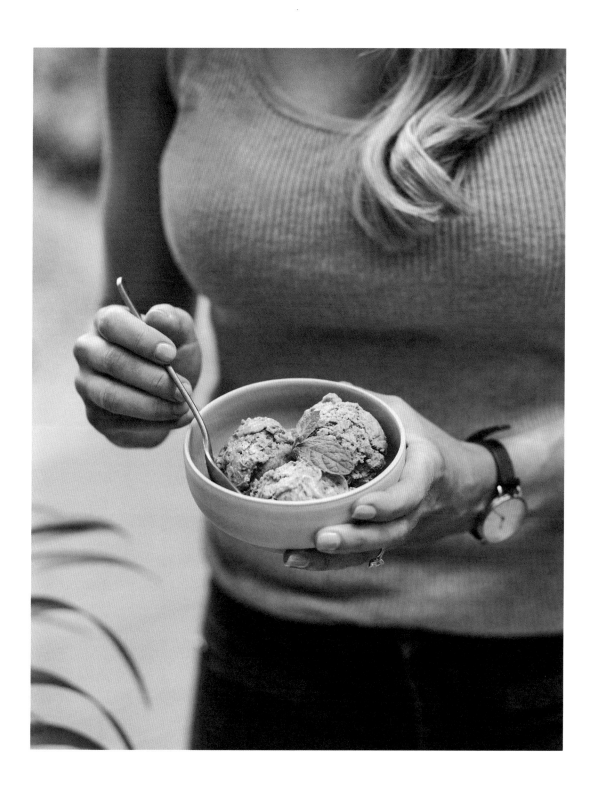

The Gut-Immune Axis

Let's face it, we're all more interested than ever before in bolstering our immunity. Whether it's staving off the common cold and winter flu, protecting ourselves against autoimmune conditions (which are on the rise), or surviving a global pandemic, we want strong defenses. "How can I boost my immunity?" is probably one of the top five questions my clients ask. (Spoiler: We don't actually want "boosted" immunity; if our immune system is overactive, it can lead to conditions such as autoimmune diseases, as I will explain.)

News headlines are forever proclaiming the next superfood or supplement that's finally going to give us super-immunity. But what we don't hear often enough is that immunity is powered by the gut. An impressive 70 percent of our immune cells actually reside in the gut, alongside our GM. And rather than sitting there rudely ignoring each other, they're in constant communication.

The GM takes on a bit of a parental role, "training" our immune cells from birth. The microbes teach our immune system what's worth reacting to (like disease-causing microbes) and what's safe (like proteins found in certain foods). Without our GM, our immunity would be pretty inefficient—think amateur athlete versus elite athlete (I know who I'd rather have on my side).

So, one of the best ways we can support our immunity is by supporting our GM—keeping it healthy by keeping our diet diverse and plant-based. The alternative? A likely disturbed GM and a poorly trained immune system that overreacts to innocent bystanders (allergies and autoimmune conditions) and underreacts to the real culprits (cold- and flu-causing viruses).

Autoimmune conditions

There are more than eighty different autoimmune conditions (where the immune system turns on itself) and, although we still have a lot to learn, there seem to be three main factors that determine whether you fall into the 5 to 8 percent of people diagnosed with one:

1. **Genetics** (we can't change these—thanks, Mom and Dad)

_____

2. **Our environment** (where we live, pollution, lifestyle)

_____

3. **Our GM** (the newly recognized player)

Our understanding of the exact role of our GM is still in its infancy, but the research is fascinating. Reduced GM diversity has been observed in a series of autoimmune conditions, as we touched on earlier, but this type of research only demonstrates that there's an association between the two, rather than one causing the other.

The first real clue that a dysbiotic GM plays a causal role in autoimmune responses was originally found in mice studies. Microbe-free mice (born into a sterile environment, so they have no GM) have been demonstrated to be protected against developing autoimmune conditions. Subsequent studies showed that transplanting the dysbiotic GM from people with autoimmune conditions into healthy mice (yes, a poop transplant, aka fecal microbiota transplant or FMT) could trigger autoimmunity, where the immune system turns on itself.

This finding has been translated into early-stage human studies, which have indicated that, in some people, FMT could be used to reverse ulcerative colitis, a type of inflammatory bowel disease that involves autoimmune activation.

Viral defense

In terms of defense against viruses, there's pretty convincing evidence that altering our GM increases our resistance, particularly when it comes to the common cold and flu (acute URTIs, or upper respiratory tract infections). In 2015, a review was conducted by a global independent network of researchers known as Cochrane, in which they looked at all the clinical trials on probiotics for acute URTIs. They found that specific probiotics could reduce the number of people getting a URTI by 47 percent, as well as reducing the duration of an episode by nearly two days if they did get one, compared to placebo. This indicates that, by giving your GM a boost, you boost your cold and flu resistance, too.

And what about *that* virus? If ever there were proof we're living in a microbial world—inside and out—it came in the form of COVID-19. Research has shown some people who contracted the virus had decreased levels of beneficial bacteria—and that their GM could predict who was more likely to become severely unwell. Another small initial study showed that a specific multi-strain probiotic (when added to standard medical care) reduced people's risk of developing respiratory failure, compared to those who just received standard care. This particular probiotic isn't commercially available yet—but fingers crossed that this will change as evidence mounts!

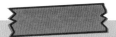

Case Study

When the World Health Organization declared a public health emergency at the end of January 2020, the severity of the new coronavirus became crystal clear. With my husband, Thomas, working on the frontline as a medical doctor, I knew he was incredibly vulnerable and I wanted to do everything I could to help support his immune system. So, I took a deep dive into the scientific literature and emerged a week later with a plan. As you may expect, it was no different from the advice I give in this book, reaffirming that what's good for the gut is good for the immune system. They really do go hand in hand.

We were both working pretty crazy hours, so I made sure the plan was as easy as possible to implement. I focused on simple but effective evidence-based actions that we could keep up for the long haul. We enjoyed quick and simple plant-powered and fiber-filled meals (which formed the basis of the Busy People menu plan on pages 122 to 123), committed to being asleep by 10 PM each night, as well as setting aside 5 minutes every evening to de-stress and reconnect, using many of the strategies outlined on page 114.

Fast forward four months to when COVID antibody tests became available to the frontline health care workers: We discovered that Thomas had actually contracted the virus. Yet he never showed one single symptom. He even commented that, despite the intensity of everything, he felt better than ever. While he was somewhat surprised, I knew the plan was grounded in science. Now, it's important to remember that this is just anecdotal evidence and is of course no guarantee, but it does support the studies so far that nourishing your gut may very well reduce your risk of becoming unwell if you do contract COVID-19.

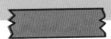

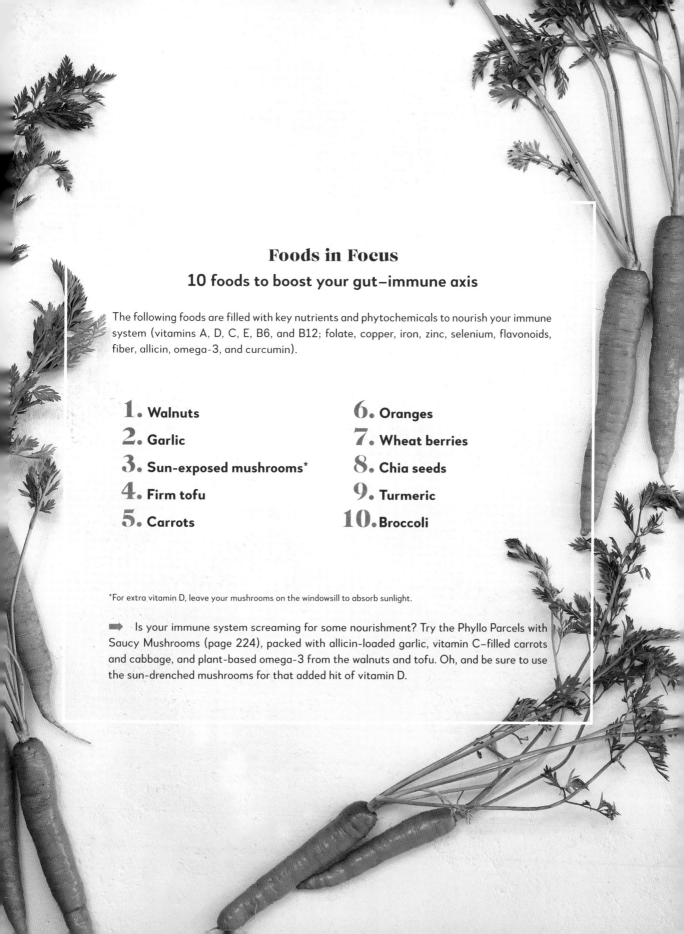

Foods in Focus

10 foods to boost your gut–immune axis

The following foods are filled with key nutrients and phytochemicals to nourish your immune system (vitamins A, D, C, E, B6, and B12; folate, copper, iron, zinc, selenium, flavonoids, fiber, allicin, omega-3, and curcumin).

1. **Walnuts**
2. **Garlic**
3. **Sun-exposed mushrooms***
4. **Firm tofu**
5. **Carrots**
6. **Oranges**
7. **Wheat berries**
8. **Chia seeds**
9. **Turmeric**
10. **Broccoli**

*For extra vitamin D, leave your mushrooms on the windowsill to absorb sunlight.

➡ Is your immune system screaming for some nourishment? Try the Phyllo Parcels with Saucy Mushrooms (page 224), packed with allicin-loaded garlic, vitamin C–filled carrots and cabbage, and plant-based omega-3 from the walnuts and tofu. Oh, and be sure to use the sun-drenched mushrooms for that added hit of vitamin D.

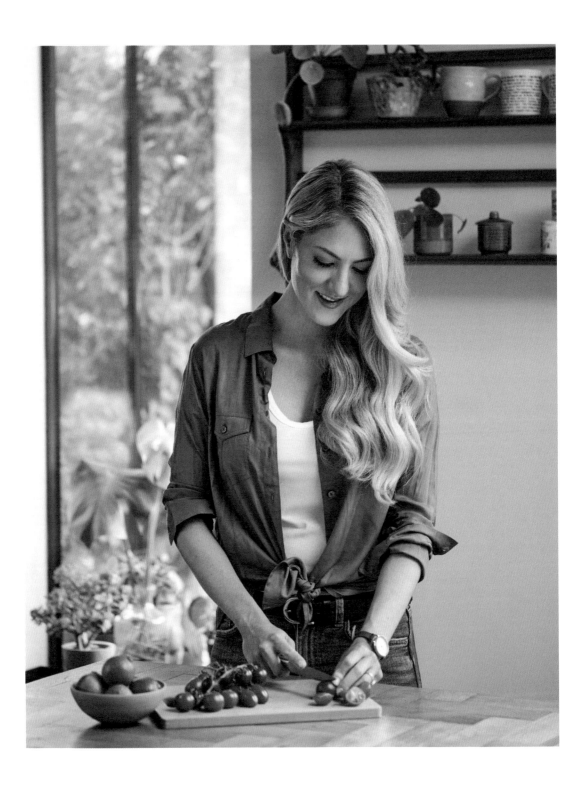

The Gut-Hormone Axis

Yet another role your all-powerful gut plays: It makes and regulates hormones. From thyroid hormones to appetite and sex hormones, our GM is proving to be quite the hormone dispenser. For a quick and clear example, remember those microbe-free mice? A study found they had abnormal sexual development and growth-hormone secretion, with fewer gender differences. Essentially, the male mice became feminized and vice versa—all because they lacked a GM to produce and help regulate their hormones.

These findings have fueled my interest in whether harnessing the power of our GM can help us better navigate the hormonal rollercoaster that is being assigned female at birth. But, guys, this area isn't exclusive to women; not only does estrogen affect people of all sexes, but a number of our gut microbes are also able to produce testosterone, and there are several parallels with estrogen balance—the clinical research just needs to catch up.

Estrogen balance

Estrogen is known as a key female hormone because it controls our reproductive cycle—from puberty to menopause—as well as each menstrual cycle. It also plays a role in the health of our heart and blood vessels, bones, breasts, skin, hair, and even our brain.

Our GM is able to influence circulating estrogen levels thanks to an enzyme it produces called beta-glucuronidase, which can turn inactive estrogen into active estrogen, recycling it from our gut back into our circulation. As a result, GM dysbiosis has been shown to negatively impact circulating estrogen levels, which can play a role in common hormonal conditions ranging from polycystic ovary syndrome, endometriosis, and infertility to breast cancer.

Equally, an abundant and diverse GM is more likely to keep estrogen levels balanced, with the potential to reduce menopausal symptoms and conditions caused by imbalances in estrogen levels. This may very well explain why in a one-year intervention study of over 17,000 menopausal women, those eating more fiber—including vegetables, fruit, and soy—experienced a 19 percent reduction in hot flashes compared to the control group.

And one systematic review (when they pool together individual trials on a topic) found that supplementing a healthy diet with specific probiotics could improve several blood markers of polycystic ovary syndrome, including hormones, compared to controls.

Insulin

It's not just about sexual health—there are hormones that control appetite, metabolism (more on those on page 72), and the hormone that regulates our blood sugar, insulin. Maintaining a healthy gut has been linked to a reduced risk of metabolic syndrome (a combination of elevated blood sugar, blood pressure, and body weight)—which, if not managed, can develop into type 2 diabetes. One very small but landmark study showed that transplanting the gut microbes from healthy, lean people (aka poop donors) into people with metabolic syndrome, was able to improve insulin sensitivity—i.e., improve their health markers. But, in case you're tempted by FMT, I must emphasize that, outside of treating life-threatening gut infections, it's not yet ready for practice given the associated risks, such as incidentally transplanting conditions like depression (as shown in mice studies). That said, all this research does support the role of nourishing our GM through diet and lifestyle to help in the management (and prevention) of a wide range of disease.

We still have so much to learn, and while it's very unlikely to be solely down to our GM, I think it's fair to say that for hormonal balance, you're going to want to keep your GM healthy.

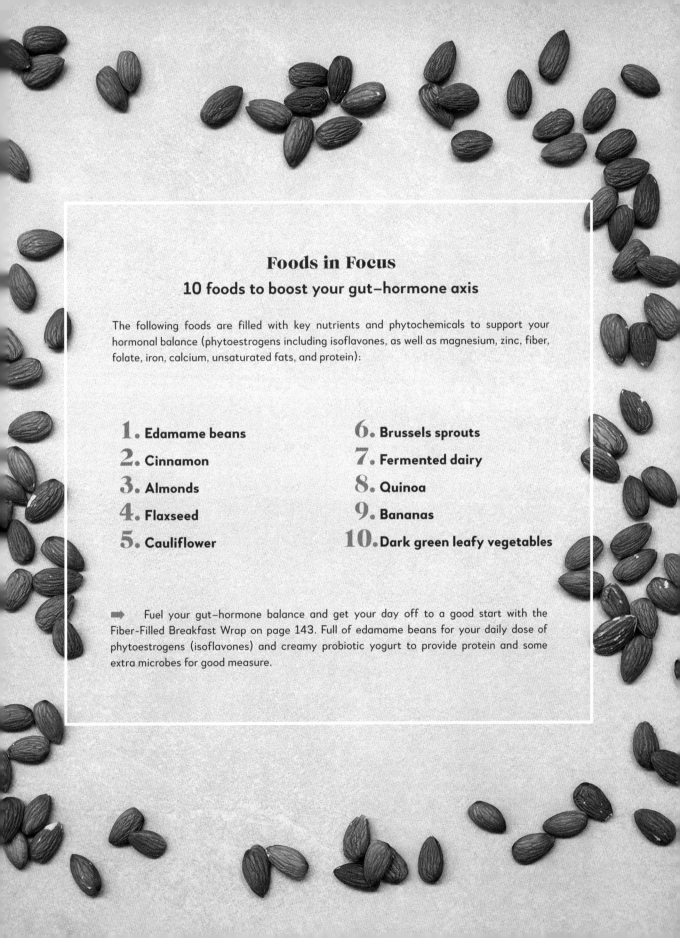

Foods in Focus
10 foods to boost your gut–hormone axis

The following foods are filled with key nutrients and phytochemicals to support your hormonal balance (phytoestrogens including isoflavones, as well as magnesium, zinc, fiber, folate, iron, calcium, unsaturated fats, and protein):

1. Edamame beans
2. Cinnamon
3. Almonds
4. Flaxseed
5. Cauliflower
6. Brussels sprouts
7. Fermented dairy
8. Quinoa
9. Bananas
10. Dark green leafy vegetables

➡ Fuel your gut–hormone balance and get your day off to a good start with the Fiber-Filled Breakfast Wrap on page 143. Full of edamame beans for your daily dose of phytoestrogens (isoflavones) and creamy probiotic yogurt to provide protein and some extra microbes for good measure.

The Gut–Metabolism Axis

We're all aware of the link between what we eat and whether we lose, gain, or maintain weight. In fact, for many people that link can become all-consuming (if you'll pardon the pun), taking all the pleasure out of eating as we struggle to balance cravings with what we think we "should" be eating. But here's some news I think you're going to like . . .

Forget calories in and out (more of that in chapter 5) or restrictive diets that are low-fat, low-carb, and so on. There's a definite link between our GM and our metabolism, and we can use this in our favor.

Our gut microbes and the chemicals they make when they digest the fiber we get from plants can impact appetite. These chemicals, such as short-chain fatty acids (SCFAs), essentially tell our body we've had enough. In turn, this halts the production of hunger hormones, such as ghrelin, and increases the "I'm full" hormones, such as leptin. This likely explains why it's often fiber intake, independent of calorie intake or type of diet, that results in healthier weight and greater dietary adherence—as shown in the appropriately named 2019 POUNDS Lost study.

And it's not just SCFA that do the "food ordering"; other chemicals produced by our GM are thought to target the reward network part of the brain, which influences our relationship with food and our tendency toward emotional eating.

Weight management

Our GM is involved in energy harvesting. Our microbes scavenge for undigested food and turn it into energy—which can be stored as fat if it's not used. But different microbes are better than others at energy harvesting and our GMs are all completely unique, which could explain why some people seem to be able to graze all day, while others feel like they just have to look at a plate to put on weight.

The gut–metabolism axis doesn't stop there. Microbes and their metabolites have been linked with "turning on" genes in your body that are related to fat distribution. They can also affect glucose and fat production and storage in the liver. Added to the fact that our microbes may influence our taste receptors and mood, it becomes pretty clear that having a higher body weight is way more complex than simply eating too much and not exercising enough. Your microbiome plays a starring role—and hey, by the end of all this research we'll probably find it's an Oscar-winning director!

If you are feeling a little defeated by these findings, remember the empowering truth of it all—much of our GM is in our control, dictated by how we feed and treat it. In fact, several studies, albeit in animals, have shown that polyphenols (plant chemicals with antioxidant powers) found in a wide range of fruit and vegetables play a prominent role in preventing weight gain by increasing metabolic rate. This mechanism appears to translate in human studies, too, since those who eat more plants tend to also have a lower body weight.

In a nutshell, feed your GM well and it's likely to keep everything else in check. So step off the scale, put down the calorie-counting calculator, and just eat more plants! That's what I advised my client Jackie, and it worked . . .

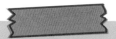

Case Study

At fifty-two years old, Jackie was going through menopause and had been dieting on and off for years—and she noticed that this behavior was now impacting her daughter's relationship with food, too. When a routine blood test found she had prediabetes, Jackie knew she had to do something.

I worked with her over four months, introducing small, practical changes. She quit calorie counting, dropped the sweeteners that were making her crave and binge on sugary foods, and shifted to the Diversity Diet.

The latter was tricky, as Jackie's years of dieting had given her an aversion to vegetables—she associated them with boring, restricted eating. I jumped at the chance to demonstrate that the Diversity Diet was anything but! Simple tricks like making batches of roast vegetables with extra virgin olive oil, smoked paprika, and rock salt (instead of her usual boiled and bland veggies) soon convinced her entire family that plants could be tasty.

I encouraged Jackie to add extra veggies to every meal and mix up her go-to pasta or rice with minimally processed whole grains such as quinoa, freekeh, and wheat berries—which she was surprised to find were actually stocked in her local supermarket—and she quickly admitted to loving these new textures and flavors. (Not sure what these whole grains are? Check out pages 100 to 101).

I showed Jackie how easy it was to add plant-based foods to regular meals, like lentils to lasagna (see the Hearty Lasagna on page 239) and quinoa to burgers (check out the Smoky Beet Burger on page 215) and naturally cutting back on meat as a result. The thing that really drove Jackie to making these long-term changes was that these were meals the entire family would enjoy and benefit from, at no extra expense (in fact, they actually saved money by buying less meat!).

We also worked on her phobia of eating fat, introducing healthy, filling options like full-fat probiotic yogurt and whole nuts. And I showed Jackie mindfulness techniques like the one on page 109, which resulted in her feeling more satisfied after each meal and so less likely to overeat.

Four months later? Her weight was down and she was fitting into those jeans that used to stare at her from the back of the wardrobe. What's more, blood tests revealed she no longer had prediabetes—reflecting the scientific evidence that you really can reverse many of these chronic conditions through diet. Jackie reported that her hot flashes had reduced, she felt less irritable, and her skin felt more hydrated. Oh, and her whole family powered through flu season, symptom-free.

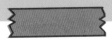

Foods in Focus
10 foods to boost your gut–metabolism axis

The following foods are filled with key nutrients and phytochemicals to support your hungry GM (fiber, including resistant starch, beta-glucan, and prebiotics; polyphenols, calcium, capsaicin, acetic acid, live microbes, iodine, and protein):

1. Natural probiotic yogurt
2. Rolled oats
3. Balsamic vinegar
4. Butter beans
5. Ginger
6. Fennel
7. Cold potato salad
8. Pistachios
9. Chile peppers
10. Grapefruit

➡ Fuel your metabolism with the Smoked Mackerel, New Potato, and Apple Salad on page 197, which contains plenty of resistant starch from the cooked and cooled potatoes, vinegar from the mustard, fermented dairy in the dressing, polyphenols from the fennel bulbs, and iodine and protein from the mackerel.

The Takeaway

There's a lot to digest (sorry, *take in*) in this chapter. But I didn't want to skim over it. And that's because I'm passionate about communicating the far-reaching benefits of improving your gut health by going plant-based. As I hope I've demonstrated here, the Diversity Diet isn't only about better digestion. It's not even just about your long-term reduced risk of many (so many!) health conditions. It's about nurturing a system of communication that affects every aspect of your health. Who knew it was so easy to make such a big impact?

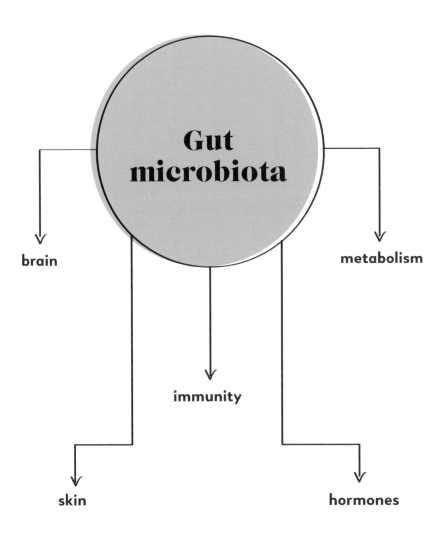

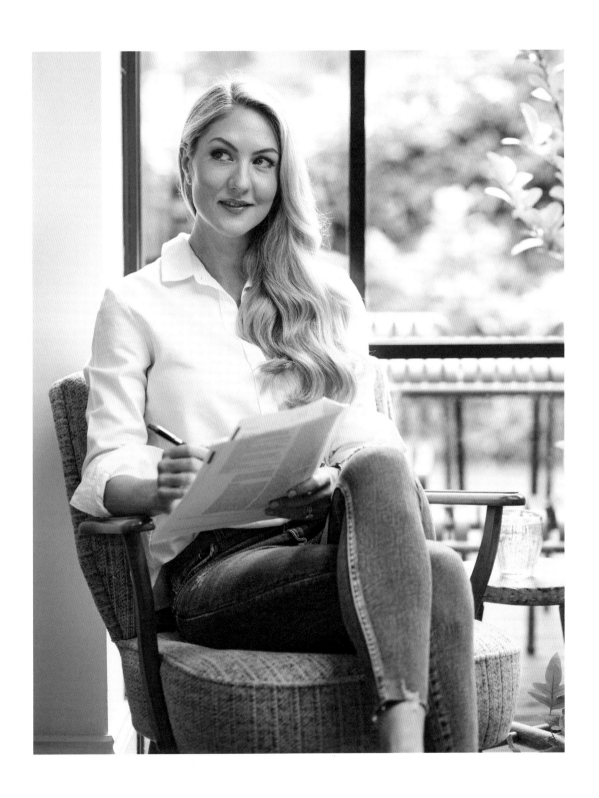

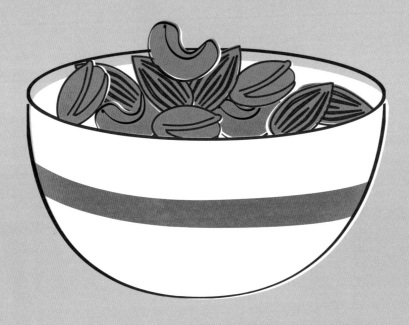

CHAPTER 5

What's Holding You Back?

Now, of course, I'm hoping you don't see any barriers to the Diversity Diet and that you're already flipping forward to the recipes, raring to get going. But if we're going to do this together, the right way, for the long term, let's really do it and leave no doubt in your mind, no lingering hang-ups, and no secret allegiance to past food fads.

In this chapter, I'm going to run through some common misconceptions about going plant-based. These are questions I often get asked by my clients, but they're easily answered. It's time to bust some myths!

If I Don't Count Calories, Won't I Gain Weight?

Ah, the great calorie conundrum. This one is a biggie, and I get that. If you've grown up with more than a passing interest in food, weight loss, or eating healthily, you might have fallen into the calorie-counting trap. It's hard not to, when the idea of balancing calories eaten versus calories burned is still the basis of most diet plans, government guidance, and even medical professionals' advice when it comes to losing weight. So why would you suddenly forget about calories and start gorging on plants?

I hear you. And I'm going to explain why I've designed the menu plans and recipes without any mention of those pesky Cs.

1. **What's listed on the package, on your food-tracking app, or online somewhere isn't as accurate as you've been led to believe.** That's because a food's calorie count is typically determined in the laboratory, simply by burning the whole food and extracting every last calorie from it. And that process is very different from what actually happens to it in our intricate digestive systems. Take almonds, for example. Human digestion studies have shown that they provide 30 percent fewer calories than what's labeled on the pack. You see, unlike in the laboratory studies, humans (and our gut microbes) don't extract every last calorie from whole plant foods. With highly processed foods, on the other hand, most of the "digesting" has already been done for us by big machines, making the calories much more accessible.

2. **Food has what's called a thermogenic effect.** That's when your body burns calories while eating and digesting. This is another reason all calories (as labeled) aren't "equal," so to speak, because your body's processing will counter some of them—and here's the important bit—depending on the *specific* food. Whole foods like fruit, vegetables, and nuts that need chewing, breaking down, and further digesting have a higher thermogenic effect than ultra-processed foods.

    One study in particular found that the calories burned digesting a meal consisting of processed foods were around 50 percent lower than those burned after a whole-food meal, despite both containing the same total carbs, fat, and protein. It might not sound enough to make a lot of difference, but over a month, a year, a lifetime? It certainly adds up.

Further research in 2019 found that people told to eat as much as they liked gained significantly more weight when given ultra-processed foods than when given unprocessed options, again even when the meals were matched for carbs, fat, and protein. This validates what I've witnessed over the past decade working with clients: that switching from processed to whole foods is a better weight-management strategy than counting "calories in."

These sorts of findings are reiterated time and time again in research and explain why we often experience a lack of satiety (that lasting feeling of fullness) after eating processed foods. You've been there, I'm sure—enjoyed a fast-food meal, felt absolutely stuffed, and then felt weirdly open to round two an hour later?

If a food has already been broken down for you, your body has less work to do and it's less satisfying. An apple takes longer to eat and is way more filling than apple sauce, which itself is more satiating than a glass of apple juice. And that's because a whole apple contains fiber and water bound up in what we call a "food matrix." The more manufacturers break a food down, often the more fiber they lose—along with that all-important food matrix.

So, if you want to feel fuller for longer and more satisfied after a meal, opt for a piece of fruit rather than a glass of juice, or rolled oats instead of quick oats—think whole plants that have been minimally "tampered" with. Understanding this and knowing why this advice really works makes those simple changes much more appealing.

3. **Food is way more than just calories.** As we saw in chapter 2, plant-based foods are packed with thousands of different nutrients and phytochemicals. Sure, a KitKat and a banana might contain similar calories—and your food-tracking app won't treat them any differently. But your body

Tip
Ditch the calorie fixation. Not only are the calorie labels inaccurate (our digestive systems are more intricate than that!) but eating whole plant foods has been shown to help with weight management, without restricting calories.

will! It'll make great use of the banana's potassium to support healthy blood pressure. Your GM will feast on the banana's prebiotic fiber. And your whole being may even get a kick from its serotonin (which you may know as the "happy hormone").

Food is also about culture, nostalgia, and family memories. I'm not about to destroy all that by asking you to put numbers on everything. That's a recipe for healthy-eating hell.

By eating a plant-based diet, we tend to feel more connected to nature and the world around us. As hippie-dippie as that sounds, the research shows this really does put us back in touch with real flavors and textures, and it's why seasonal eating has become such a trend in recent years.

If you're still not convinced that there's no need to fixate on calories when upping your plant intake, and if weight management is your main concern when thinking about how to improve your diet, here's something that is sure to put those thoughts to bed. A meta-analysis (when researchers pull together the results of individual studies—fifteen, in this case) has shown that plant-based eating can result in a significant reduction in body weight, without any restrictions on portion size or calorie intake. The proof is in the pudding.

But I'll definitely Put On Weight If I Gorge on Nuts and Avocado . . .

There are certain foods I call "halo foods" because they've hit the headlines for being healthy and now are everywhere—in recipes, on café menus, all over Instagram—to signal that people are making "good" food choices. Indeed, they *are* good for us, but that doesn't mean we should eat them to excess and to the exclusion of other plants.

Peanut butter, I'm looking at you. Yes, you're damn tasty. Yes, you're a valuable source of plant protein, healthy fats, vitamins, and minerals, and a decent slow-release source of energy. But you're not the only healthy plant food out there.

Another huge one is smashed avocado. I'm on to you, too. I know you're a good source of unsaturated fat, fiber, potassium, and folate—but you're not the only one. There are plenty more healthy foods not getting attention thanks to you hogging the limelight.

It all comes back to the D-word: *diversity*. Sure, have your PB and avo, but mix it up. Get those plant points to 30 and beyond (including a portion of nuts or seeds each day, see page 15).

If you do find yourself feeling "out of control" and eating one plant-based food or group much more than any other (which can be quite common, especially if you're coming from a restrictive diet), it's worth exploring the mindful-eating exercise on page 109. It's all about getting back in tune with your body's hunger and satiety signals.

Won't I Be Protein-Deficient If I Eat Only Plants?

First, let's recap chapter 1. This is about being plant-*based*, not plants-*only*. Animal products, if you want them, are definitely still on the menu. Vegetarians, famously, have a reduced risk of all-cause mortality (death for any reason), but studies also show the same is true of diets that simply place more of an emphasis on plants.

Second, plants contain protein, too. I'm going to say the D-word again, because so long as your focus is on *diversity*, you'll likely be getting all the protein building blocks (amino acids) you need. And if you're talking about building your muscle mass to achieve a fitness goal, an increasing number of professional athletes are vegan, reaffirming that protein from plants is more than sufficient in supporting our bodies when training. For more on this, flip back to page 37.

I'm Vegan, So I'm There Already, Right?

You'd be forgiven for thinking that you've already ticked all the healthy boxes by following a vegan diet, but the truth is that simply excluding animal products isn't what will support your GM and therefore your overall health. Instead, you need to look at what sort of plant-based foods make up your vegan diet. Remember that plant-based diet index on page 28? The key is how processed and diverse your plants are.

As vegan diets have moved into the mainstream, food manufacturers have responded by making more and more convenience foods for "vegans on the go." I'm talking fake ham, fake hot dogs, meatless sausages, vegan cheese, you name it. While this might seem like progress, these kinds of ultra-processed food are not what your GM needs. Soy protein, in particular, is used to make many meat-substitute products. But to get to that malleable product with a meaty texture, it has to go through many processes to transform from its original life as whole soybeans—not to mention the food additives, several of which are currently under investigation as GM disruptors. These sorts of foods are also often high in salt (which, in excess, can negatively impact our GM).

So, although you might be following a vegan diet and feel pretty healthy in that decision, highly processed meat alternatives are definitely not doing as much for you as their whole-food counterparts.

What You *Can't* Get from Plants

While we can get a huge amount of the nutrients we need from eating plants, going vegan can make it a little more challenging to meet your body's needs for specific things. This is because animal foods are the main and often most easily absorbed source of several of the essential nutrients, including calcium, iron, zinc, vitamin B12, iodine, selenium, choline, and long-chain omega-3 fatty acids (DHA and EPA).

This is why I generally recommend a plant-*based* diet rather than an exclusively vegan diet. But if you do want to take the exclusive approach, by all means go ahead. I generally recommend my vegan clients supplement their diet with B12 (at least 10 micrograms a day) and algae-derived DHA and EPA fatty acids (around 250 milligrams a day), and make a concerted effort to get those missing nutrients from foods like nutritional yeast, fortified plant-based milks, Brazil nuts, nori, walnuts, flaxseed, and seeded sourdough.

Interestingly, our GM actually can make its own B12. This is why there's a subset of vegans who don't need to take supplements. However, most people's GMs don't make enough, so it's best to be safe and up your intake, especially if you don't have access to testing.

Plant-Based Food Is Too Expensive and Hard to Find

I'm not denying that there are plenty of stores where a week's worth of plant-based groceries could cost you a month's wages. But despite what they'd love you to believe, you certainly don't need to shop in those places to follow the Diversity Diet. Everything in this book is available from your mainstream supermarket of choice, your local farmers market, or your corner shop; and lots of it you can even grow in your garden. The bottom line is that plant-based diversity can be easy *and* affordable—just stick to my four tips on page 87. Not only have they helped many of my patients on a budget, they're also what I lived by when I first moved to London and struggled to make ends meet.

You don't need to take my word for it either. A study looking at the costs of going plant-based showed that, despite the participants' initial perception, the cost of their weekly grocery basket actually went down over time.

Cost-Saving Tips

1. Buy fruit and vegetables in season.

The recipes in this book are very much adaptable by season. If it says pomegranate (winter fruit) but you're making it in summer, use strawberries instead—you can't really go wrong. How do you know which fruit and vegetables are in season? The price! They're around half the price when in season. You can also check out the seasonality lists on my website theguthealthdoctor.com.

2. Bulk out your meat dishes with legumes.

The ultimate cost-saver, whether you soak and cook them from scratch or opt for canned. Even the "fancier" protein options, such as tofu, are cheaper than meat.

3. Don't let your produce go bad!

Many of the recipes in this book are labeled with a "Fridge Raid" icon (see page 116). This is your opportunity to use up any wilting veggies or bruised fruit. And don't forget about the freezer. If you buy in bulk, particularly when plants are in season, utilize the freezer as your ultimate preserver. For most vegetables, just blanch them in boiling water for a few minutes before chileng and freezing. Fruit, on the other hand, is ready to go straight in! The exception being fruit and veggies with high water content, like watermelon and cucumber. These are best eaten fresh.

4. Take your own snacks when out and about.

This means that you don't have to succumb to the $3 "vegan" energy balls when hunger strikes. I've got a recipe on page 144 that costs less than 20 cents per ball to make, and you can keep them in the freezer for months.

I Can Get All the Nutrients I Need–without All the Cooking–by Taking Supplements

I'm afraid I hear this a lot, but it isn't entirely true. You remember Harry from chapter 2, who thought he could hit his daily plant quota with his meal-replacement shakes? It didn't work for him, and it's unlikely to work for you. These shakes claim to provide all the fat, carbs, protein, vitamins, and minerals you need each day. But as you know by now, real food offers so much more nutrition, not to mention flavor (and where's that all-important food matrix in liquid food?). So, let Silicon Valley supply your tech, not your nutrition.

Dietary supplements are big business. From single vitamins and minerals to multi-formulations and blends for specific purposes (brain power, digestion, sleep), you can buy them all in capsule form. And sometimes, undoubtedly, they're helpful. Vitamin D, for example, is a must for everyone living in countries with limited sunlight exposure during the winter months, and there are several cases where I recommend specific supplements (such as probiotics, fiber supplements, and peppermint capsules) in my clinic. But these really should be taken on a case-by-case basis, and the formulations are backed by clinical trials. The chances are you don't need most, if any, of those bottles of vitamins that line the shelves of high-street pharmacies, no matter how convincing their "boost your energy" and "strengthen your nails" claims are.

Not only can they be a waste of money, we also know that some isolated nutrients can be harmful in high doses or interact with other medications (one example is vitamin E). If you take a range of formulations and don't study all the labels closely, you could easily be ingesting too much of certain vitamins or minerals. On the other hand, it's hard to overdose on single nutrients in whole foods, the way Mother Nature packages them. Food contains what you need, in safe portions, which is why eating a diverse diet is the most effective and fail-safe way to give your body what it needs.

Will I Have to Give Up My Favorite Foods?

This isn't an all-or-nothing approach. As I said at the beginning—it's about enriching, not restricting. I don't want anyone to give up something they love. There's no way I'm going to live my best life without having white chocolate!

That's the beauty of the Diversity Diet: It's about adding in plants for your microbes to enjoy, alongside your taste buds' favorites, which is why I designed my crave-busting Pistachio Berry Bursts (page 284).

Rather than giving up and feeling deprived, you'll soon find that by adding in plants you'll discover new flavors and recipes that will have your taste buds wishing you'd started eating this way much earlier. Many of the recipes in this book will become your new favorites— and because they're so filling, you'll naturally feel more satisfied, with fewer cravings.

The earlier you start with children the better, too, so be sure to give my menu plan for the whole family a try (see page 120) and you'll have the kids on board before you know it. But rest assured, there's always room for your old recipe favorites, and you may even be enticed to make a few tweaks after reading chapter 6. Plant-based is tasty and fun!

Bloating, Cramps . . . Gas! I'm Sorry, but Too Much of the Plant Stuff Just Doesn't Agree with Me

This is a really important conversation to have, because all too often I see people in my clinic who have experienced such severe gut symptoms that they have stripped most of the fiber out of their diet—and are nervous to add it back in. One of the most common questions I get asked is: "Why can I tolerate meat, fish, and refined carbs like white rice, but not vegetables or whole grains?"

The simple answer is that these foods, unlike high-fiber foods such as vegetables, are mostly digested by human enzymes higher up in your gut. They don't rely on your GM to digest them. For the "smooth" (symptomless) digestion of fiber, however, you need two things:

1. Microbes that are equipped with enough enzymes to digest the fiber you're eating.
If over a short period of time you go from a very low-fiber diet to one that has loads of fiber, your digestion is unlikely to feel smooth—most people can expect bloating, a change in pooping habits, and so on, as the body adjusts. As we discussed in chapter 3, this is partly because your microbe profile hasn't yet adapted to reflect the foods you're giving it (picture a new café that is overwhelmed by the demand in its first few weeks, but then hires more staff to handle all the customers). It's also worth keeping in mind that a little gas and bloating is the sign of a well-fed GM—i.e., it's completely normal and isn't to be feared.

Try this: A slow introduction of plant diversity, to give your microbes time to assemble all the right "tools" to get to work on that great fiber. That could mean starting by adding half a normal portion of plants per day. Try half a piece of fruit or ¼ cup of legumes per sitting, or stick to just one of the high-fiber recipes in this book per day. If your gut is more sensitive, you might want to start with a quarter of a portion and work up to half and then a whole portion over several months. For more tips, turn to page 112.

2. A relaxed gut.
If you have an uptight gut—meaning you're stressed (which can be unconscious for some), or perhaps your gut itself is stressed after an infection (such as food poisoning or gastritis)—your gut wall isn't very efficient at absorbing the gas and other chemicals that are produced by your GM during fiber digestion. Instead of the gas being efficiently absorbed across your gut wall and into your bloodstream (where it's then breathed out through your lungs), it can get trapped in your gut, causing those symptoms of bloating, cramps, and flatulence. This can explain why some days you might be fine with a specific higher-fiber food, but other days it feels like a total disaster. The annoying truth is that it's not always about the food; it has to do with the state of your gut–brain axis.

Try this: Alongside the slow fiber introduction described above, find time to de-stress with some yoga, mindfulness, or whatever else brings your mind and body into a relaxed state. The science shows that it really can help your digestion. For more tips on this, turn to pages 109 to 111.

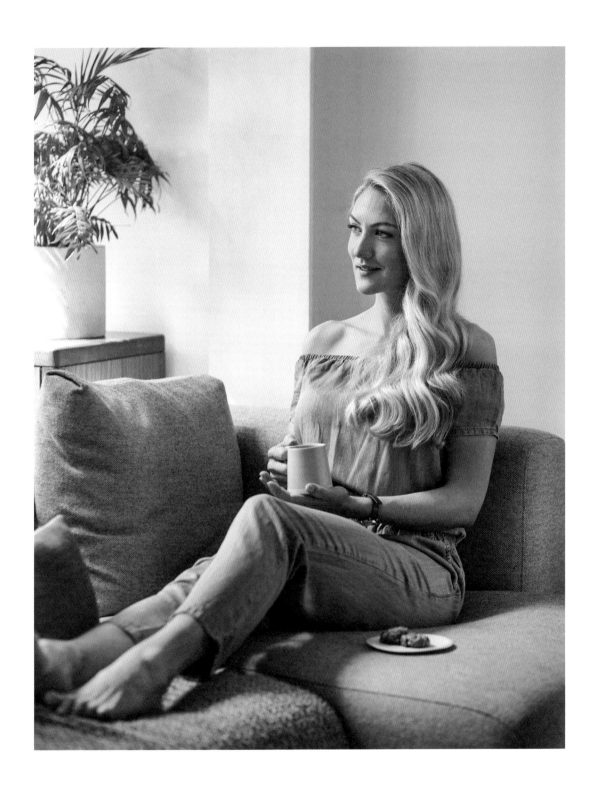

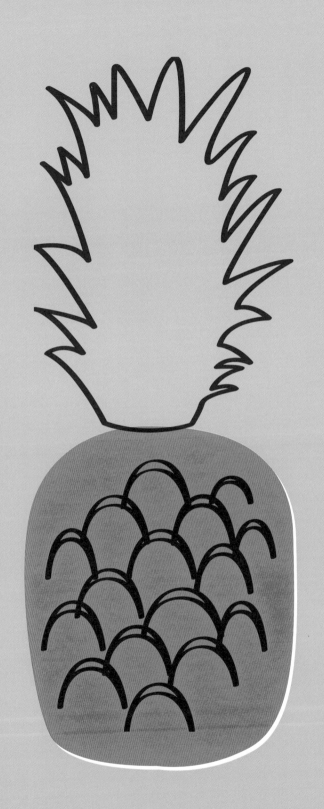

CHAPTER 6

The Diversity Diet Toolkit

Ready to get going? I hope that by now you're at least tempted to join the Diversity Diet revolution. The next (and final) step is to show you that making the transition is easy—and dare I say even a little exciting—as we take your taste buds on a culinary adventure. Sure, knowledge is key, and understanding why you're making a change will underpin your motivation and commitment. But I'm also a big believer in practical advice. It's about that extra helping hand to make the transition to a more nutritious and delicious way of eating. In this chapter, you'll find everything you need to take that next step—including tailored meal plans and a 28-day plant point challenge that makes getting all of your plant points fun. Think of it as your Diversity Diet toolkit.

My Top Diversity Hacks

Looking for easy ways to get your weekly plant points to 30 and beyond? Why not give one of these **quick switches**, **habit formers**, and **easy adds** a try each week?

Quick switches:

1. Peckish? Swap chips for a handful of toasted nuts or seeds, or try saving your potato or butternut squash peelings to roast in the oven for a crispy snack (see my sweet potato gnocchi recipe on page 246). It's a great way to reduce your food waste, too!

2. If you're making a fruit crumble, substitute a third of the flour with oats and another third with ground almonds (check out page 287 for my gut-loving Naked Fruit Crumble).

3. Don't just add kidney beans to your chili; use mixed beans for greater diversity.

4. Switch your single piece of fruit for half a cup of mixed berries (fresh or frozen).

5. Craving crackers and dip? Sub out those plain boring crackers for a seedy selection (check out my Seedy Cracker Duo on page 177) or veggie sticks such as green beans, sugar snap peas, and asparagus—no chopping necessary!

Habit formers:

1. Every time you go to serve up a meal at home, stop and think, *What could I add?* Chop a banana over your granola (see page 145 for my DIY Plant-Packed Granola), add some sprouts to your sandwich, slice a tomato onto your plate—every bit counts.

2. Are you a habit shopper? We all do it! Once a month, allow an extra thirty minutes in the supermarket to browse the plant-food aisles. You may be surprised by the different varieties available. Or seek out a new farmers market or farm shop to visit, to give you some inspiration.

3. Stock up on frozen veggies and fruit—so when you've got nothing fresh left, it doesn't matter. For extra diversity, buy mixed bags of both.

4. Whether you're eating out or cooking at home, aim to try a different cuisine once a week— it'll introduce you to new plants and flavors.

5. Consider signing up for a local CSA (community supported agriculture) vegetable box if you have access to one, as each delivery gives you different plants and encourages you to try new things.

Easy adds:

1. Most, if not all, dishes will benefit from the addition of some herbs or spices, which also add some extra phytochemicals to your meal. Keep your dried herb and spice jars out where you can see them, so you don't forget to sprinkle a few into each meal.

2. No casserole, stew, risotto, or pie is complete without one more vegetable than the recipe calls for—it can be as simple as adding a can of lentils or chickpeas (think of the cost saving, too).

3. Add mixed seeds to a shaker and add a sprinkle to cereal, yogurt, smoothies, and salads. Seeds work as a tasty, crunchy topper for scrambled eggs, avocado toast, or soup.

4. Grow your own fresh herbs— you only need a windowsill—and add them in handfuls to salads. Think of them as leaves packed with plant goodness, rather than just for flavoring—use them generously and go big on taste.

5. Try a new whole grain or legume in an old-favorite recipe. Not familiar with all the different types of legumes? Turn to my guide on pages 102 to 103.

Wheel of Diversity

This wheel shows just a glimpse of the wide array of options within the Super Six: whole grains, fruits, vegetables, nuts and seeds, legumes, and herbs and spices. We really are spoiled for choice! I'm sure there are some foods here you already have as a regular part of your diet and others you haven't had for months or perhaps have never tried. Bottom line: This wheel isn't exhaustive, it's for inspiration—and I bet you can add to it!

Not sure what's in season? Head to my website (theguthealthdoctor.com) where there are lists of what's at its best (and also most affordable) by season.

Whole grains
- Buckwheat
- Barley
- Amaranth
- Corn
- Farro
- Freekeh
- Millet
- Oats
- Quinoa
- Rye
- Sorghum
- Spelt
- Teff
- Wheat
- Wheat berries
- Wild rice

Herbs and spices
- Black pepper
- Cardamom
- Chile
- Chives
- Cilantro/Coriander
- Cinnamon
- Cumin
- Fennel
- Ginger
- Mint
- Mustard seeds
- Nutmeg
- Oregano
- Paprika
- Parsley
- Rosemary
- Turmeric

Legumes
- Adzuki beans
- Black beans
- Black-eyed peas
- Borlotti/cranberry beans
- Broad beans/fava beans
- Butter beans
- Cannellini beans
- Chickpeas
- Edamame/soybeans
- Kidney beans
- Lentils
- Lupin beans
- Mung beans
- Navy beans
- Pinto beans
- Yellow split peas

Nuts and seeds
- Almonds
- Brazil nuts
- Cashews
- Chia seeds
- Flaxseeds
- Hemp seeds
- Hazelnuts
- Pecans
- Peanuts
- Pine nuts
- Pistachios
- Poppy seeds
- Pumpkin seeds
- Sesame seeds
- Sunflower seeds
- Watermelon seed
- Walnuts

Vegetables
- Zucchini
- Sweet potato
- Spinach
- Peppers
- Mushrooms
- Leeks
- Jackfruit
- Green beans
- Eggplant
- Celery
- Cauliflower
- Carrots
- Brussels sprouts
- Broccoli
- Bok choy
- Beets
- Asparagus
- Artichokes

Fruit
- Apples
- Apricots
- Bananas
- Blueberries
- Dates
- Figs
- Kiwi
- Limes
- Mango
- Melon
- Oranges
- Peaches
- Pears
- Pineapple
- Plums
- Pomegranate
- Raspberries

Your Plant-Based Shopping List

Increasing your diversity does require you to get a little experimental, inquisitive, and imaginative when you hit the shops. I heartily encourage you to shop with the seasons and buy what you like when it comes to fresh produce. But when it comes to those pantry staples, the following is a good guide to making sure you're recipe-ready for a plant-based feast.

Flours and powders

- ○ Almond flour/almond meal
- ○ Baking powder
- ○ Cocoa powder
- ○ Rye flour
- ○ Spelt flour
- ○ Whole wheat flour

Whole grains

- ○ Barley
- ○ Buckwheat/soba noodles
- ○ Freekeh
- ○ Mixed whole grains
- ○ Quinoa
- ○ Rolled oats
- ○ Sourdough bread
- ○ Wheat berries
- ○ Whole wheat pasta

Fruits and sweeteners

- ○ Coconut flakes
- ○ Cranberries
- ○ Dark chocolate

- ○ Dried apricots
- ○ Dried mango
- ○ Dried figs
- ○ Frozen mixed berries
- ○ Goji berries
- ○ Medjool dates
- ○ Raisins

Nuts and seeds

- ○ 100 percent nut butter
- ○ Brazil nuts
- ○ Cashews
- ○ Chia seeds
- ○ Flaxseed meal
- ○ Hazelnuts
- ○ Mixed seeds
- ○ Mixed unsalted nuts
- ○ Pecans
- ○ Pine nuts
- ○ Pistachios
- ○ Sesame seeds
- ○ Tahini
- ○ Walnuts

Canned/preserved vegetables

○ Canned whole tomatoes/tomato puree

○ Capers

○ Frozen mixed vegetables

○ Frozen peas

○ Jackfruit

○ Jalapeños

○ Marinated artichokes

○ Nori seaweed

○ Olives

○ Pickled vegetables

○ Roasted peppers

○ Sun-dried tomatoes

Herbs and spices

○ Cinnamon

○ Cumin

○ Curry powder

○ Garlic

○ Ginger

○ Mixed herbs

○ Nutmeg

○ Red pepper flakes

○ Rosemary

○ Smoked paprika

○ Thyme

○ Turmeric

○ Vanilla extract

○ Vegetable stock

Condiments

○ Coconut milk and cream

○ Dijon mustard

○ Harissa paste

○ Miso paste

○ Nutritional yeast

○ Soy sauce/tamari

○ Worcestershire sauce

Legumes

○ Black beans

○ Butter beans

○ Chickpeas

○ Kidney beans

○ Mixed beans, in water

○ Silken tofu

○ Pretty much one of every can on the shelf!

Oils and vinegars

○ Apple cider vinegar

○ Balsamic vinegar

○ Extra virgin olive oil

○ Sesame oil

Tip

Although it works out cheaper to buy dried legumes, the prep required is a barrier for most. Treat your microbes and go for the cans! Just be sure to pick up the ones in water, not in brine or sauce.

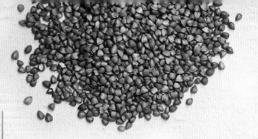

Meet and Greet: Whole Grains

From the bread you eat and the flour you bake with, to the pasta and rice that accompanies your dinner, it's so easy to get into a rut with whole grains. If you tend to rely on the same old staples (like wheat, rice, and oats), it's time to get acquainted with some of the other deserving options, and learn why they're so great and how you can use them. You may be surprised to find that most of these whole grains are available in major supermarkets at no extra cost.

Buckwheat

Despite its name, it's not actually related to wheat. Most commonly found in its whole grain form (often called a groat), it's also made into flour and noodles (soba).

- **Nutrition need-to-know:** One serving (¼ cup/ 40 g raw) delivers 4 g fiber, 6 g protein, and nearly 25 percent of your daily magnesium needs. A good source of rutin, a polyphenol that packs quite the antioxidant punch and is linked to improved heart health. It's also gluten-free.

- **Flavor profile and where to use it:** With a robust and earthy taste, the whole grains make a good oatmeal substitute, although soba noodles in a rich soup are my favorite way to eat buckwheat.

- **Find it in:** Stir-Fry Adventures (pages 218 to 220)

Red rice

A variety of rice that is naturally colored red by the polyphenol anthocyanin.

- **Nutrition need-to-know:** One serving (¼ cup/ 45 g raw) delivers 5 g fiber (four times higher than standard white rice) and 4 g protein. High in the polyphenol anthocyanin, which is linked with brain health. It's also gluten-free.

- **Flavor profile and where to use it:** Nutty flavor that works well as a substitute in most savory rice dishes, excluding risotto, given its non-glutinous texture.

- **Find it in:** Fried Quinoa with Hoisin Drizzle (see note on page 273)

Rye

A close relative of wheat (found in bread, pasta, and couscous) and barley (found in beer, malted products, some multigrain breads, and soups), rye is often made into flakes (for hot cereal) and flour.

- **Nutrition need-to-know:** One serving (¼ cup/ 40 g raw) delivers 6 g fiber and 4 g of protein. Whole grain rye has been shown to have less impact on blood sugar compared to other whole grains, due to its high levels of viscous arabinoxylan fiber.

- **Flavor profile and where to use it:** With a strong, slightly sour yet earthy taste, rye flour makes a great substitute for wheat flour in savory baked goods such as bread and muffins. Best known as the whole grain behind pumpernickel bread.

- **Find it in:** Seedy Cracker Duo (page 177)

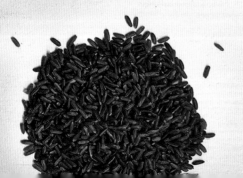

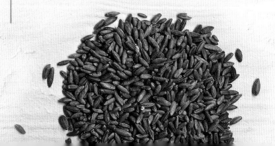

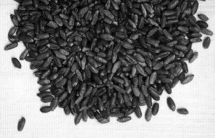

Freekeh

An ancient type of wheat that's roasted and rubbed to create its flavor.

- **Nutrition need-to-know:** One serving (¼ cup/ 40 g raw) delivers 4 g fiber, 5 g protein, and 15 percent of your daily iron needs, plus the plant chemicals lutein and zeaxanthin, which are linked to eye health.

- **Flavor profile and where to use it:** A fluffy and chewy whole grain with a signature smoky flavor. Ideal for adding texture to soups and salads. Try it in place of couscous.

- **Find it in**: Roasted Veggie and Freekeh Salad (page 196)

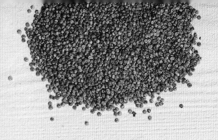

Quinoa

Technically a pseudograin, this is really a seed, but it's prepared and eaten similarly to a whole grain. There are three main types: white, black, and red.

- **Nutrition need-to-know:** One serving (¼ cup/ 40 g raw) delivers 3 g fiber, 6 g protein, and nearly 20 percent of your daily folate needs. Quinoa is one of the few plant foods that serves up a complete protein, offering all essential amino acids in a healthy balance. It's also gluten-free.

- **Flavor profile and where to use it:** A mild flavor with a firm texture makes it easy to include at breakfast, lunch, or dinner. Ideal for breakfast bowls and saucy dishes. Try it in place of rice.

- **Find it in:** Smoky Beet Burger (page 215)

Spelt

An ancient type of wheat, also known as dinkel wheat.

- **Nutrition need-to-know:** One serving (¼ cup/ 40 g raw) delivers 5 g fiber, 6 g protein, and over 50 percent of your daily manganese needs (an essential mineral for the normal workings of your brain and nervous system).

- **Flavor profile and where to use it:** Hearty and slightly nutty, spelt adds more depth of flavor than standard wheat. An easy substitute for standard wheat flour in most baking, both sweet and savory.

- **Find it in:** Butternut Muffins (page 191)

Wheat berries

The whole wheat kernel with the food matrix intact, including all three layers: bran (fiber), germ (the nutrient-packed core containing B vitamins and healthy fats) and endosperm (a starchy component containing protein). Whole wheat flour also contains each of these elements—they've just been ground up. Processed white flour just contains the endosperm.

- **Nutrition need-to-know:** One serving (¼ cup/ 45 g raw) delivers 6 g fiber, 6 g protein, and 15 percent of your daily zinc needs.

- **Flavor profile and where to use them:** Sweet, creamy yet nutty flavor. The berries hold their shape and keep their chewy bite, which makes them ideal as a barley substitute in soups, for textured rice dishes, and baked into bread to add texture.

- **Find it in:** Korean-Inspired Stir-Fry (page 220)

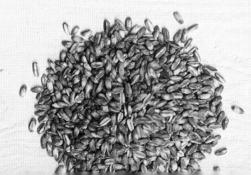

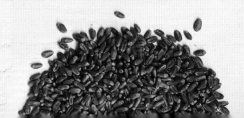

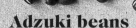

Meet and Greet: Legumes

Generally speaking, legumes are any plants that grow in pods—including beans and pulses, which are the edible seeds within the pods. Pulses were some of the first crops cultivated, as far back as 11,000 years ago. All these legumes are widely available and affordable in cans, or even cheaper if you buy them dried, then soak and cook them. They're also one of the most sustainable sources of protein: good for you, your microbes, and the planet, and naturally gluten-free.

Adzuki beans

Also known as red mung beans, these are popular in Japan in both sweet and savory dishes.

- **Nutrition need-to-know:** One serving (½ cup/ 115 g cooked) delivers 8 g fiber, 9 g protein, and nearly 20 percent of your daily zinc needs. They also pack quite the polyphenol punch, including flavanols, which are linked to skin health.

- **Flavor profile and where to use them:** Subtly sweet and versatile, these work well in most dishes, including soups, casseroles, and chili. For something sweet, blend them with your natural sweetener of choice (I love dates) to make the sweet Japanese red bean paste, anko.

- **Find them in:** Leafy Taco Wraps (page 187)

Butter beans

The name says it all—blending these creamy beans makes the perfect substitute for butter, without all that saturated fat.

- **Nutrition need-to-know:** One serving (½ cup/ 95 g cooked) delivers 7 g fiber, 7 g protein, and over 20 percent of your daily manganese needs.

- **Flavor profile and where to use them:** Soft and buttery, these work well in stews, where they can soak up all the flavors. Or try blending them as you would chickpeas to make a winning hummus or mayonnaise replacement.

- **Find them in:** Crispy Bacon-Shrooms with Creamy Butter Bean Hummus (page 146)

Cannellini beans

Also known as white kidney beans because of their shape, these originate in Italy.

- **Nutrition need-to-know:** One serving (½ cup/ 110 g cooked) delivers 6 g fiber and 7 g protein. Like most legumes, they're a notable source of iron, but remember to combine them with a source of vitamin C, such as peppers or tomatoes, to help them reach their iron-delivering potential.

- **Flavor profile and where to use them:** With a fluffy texture and slightly nutty flavor, these go perfectly in stir-fries and salads. They also make a great sub for short-cut pasta in dishes such as minestrone soup and are delicious added to mac and cheese.

- **Find them in:** Creamy Beans with "Meaty" Jackfruit (page 245)

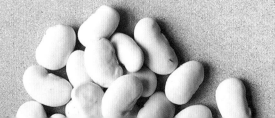

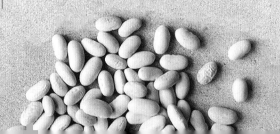

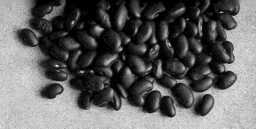
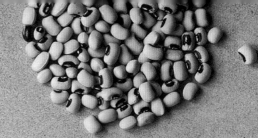

Black beans

A staple food in Central and South America that, when eaten with rice, blunts the blood sugar rise compared to eating just rice.

- **Nutrition need-to-know:** One serving (½ cup/ 85 g cooked) delivers 8 g fiber, 8 g protein, and 15 percent of your daily magnesium needs. They're also one of the highest sources of polyphenols within the legume family, thanks to the anthocyanins (also found in blueberries) that are largely responsible for their rich black color.

- **Flavor profile and where to use them:** Floury and mild in flavor, they make a great replacement for flour in moist, gluten-free chocolate brownies and muffins. They also go well in spicy savory dishes, including burritos.

- **Find them in:** Muffin in a Mug (page 140)

Black-eyed peas

These visually distinct beans resemble eyes, making them a hit with kids. In the South, eating them on New Year's Day is thought to bring prosperity.

- **Nutrition need-to-know:** One serving (½ cup/ 85 g cooked) delivers 6 g fiber, 7 g protein, and over 40 percent of our daily folate needs (not including during pregnancy).

- **Flavor profile and where to use them:** Creamy and earthy, these make a great addition to any dish with rice or couscous. Or fry them in olive oil with garlic, onion, and chopped tomatoes as they do in Syria and Lebanon. Yum!

- **Find them in:** Leafy Taco Wraps (page 187)

Navy beans

Popular as baked beans, they are also one of the best sources of fiber in the legume family.

- **Nutrition need-to-know:** One serving (½ cup/ 90 g cooked) delivers 10 g fiber, 8 g protein, and nearly 20 percent of your thiamine (vitamin B1) needs.

- **Flavor profile and where to use them:** A little on the bland side, these beans have made their mark thanks to their excellent ability to absorb the flavors of a dish. This makes them ideal to soak up saucy dishes such as tomatoes in baked beans, and stews.

- **Find them in:** Green Pea and "Ham" Soup (page 232)

Pinto beans

One of the most popular bean varieties, you may not recognize these in their dried form, as they lose their specks once cooked.

- **Nutrition need-to-know:** One serving (½ cup/ 85 g cooked) delivers 8 g fiber and 8 g protein. They are particularly rich in kaempferol, a flavonoid associated with impressive anti-inflammatory benefits and lowering cholesterol.

- **Flavor profile and where to use them:** Soft with a mild nutty flavor, these versatile beans are often eaten whole, mashed, or fried. I recommend them mashed with roasted garlic and onion as an addicting spread.

- **Find them in:** Baked Sweet Potato Trio (page 198)

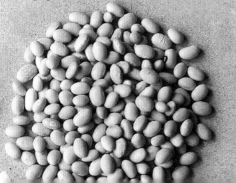
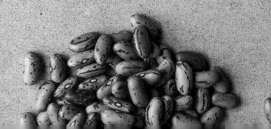

Cooking Tips

- **Boiling, steaming, baking, sautéing, frying . . .** there are many different ways to prepare your plants. I encourage you to mix it up, because all of these methods create different flavors. To maximize nutrient retention, use as little water as possible when poaching and boiling, and don't peel veggies until after cooking (better still, don't peel them at all, for more fiber).

- **In a rush?** Steam your root vegetables in the microwave with a splash of water to soften them before baking. This reduces baking time by around 20 minutes.

- **Roasted vegetables are so versatile,** so if you're going to the effort of roasting, make a double or even triple batch as they last in the fridge for up to five days and make a great addition to most meals (wraps, salads, and sandwiches included) and a great snack (try my One-Minute Sweet Potato Slider on page 304).

- **Learning to love a new plant?** Be sure to dress it up! See pages 172 to 175 for some of my favorite dips and pages 218 to 220 for my favorite stir-fries.

- **Seasoning your plants is quick and tasty,** and it adds even more plant goodness. Here are some of my favorite flavor combos:

Legumes	Stir fries (see pages 218 to 220 for my top stir-fry recipes)	Salad dressings	Breads and crackers	Fruits
✓ cayenne	✓ basil	✓ basil	✓ caraway	✓ allspice
✓ cumin	✓ bay leaves	✓ celery seed	✓ cardamom	✓ cardamom
✓ curry powder	✓ celery seed	✓ chives	✓ cinnamon	✓ cinnamon
✓ parsley	✓ curry powder	✓ dill	✓ coriander	✓ cloves
✓ red pepper flakes	✓ dill	✓ fennel	✓ cumin	✓ coriander
✓ rosemary	✓ garlic	✓ horseradish	✓ dill	✓ ginger
✓ sage	✓ ginger	✓ mint	✓ orange peel	✓ mint
✓ thyme	✓ oregano	✓ mustard	✓ oregano	✓ star anise
	✓ parsley	✓ oregano	✓ rosemary	
	✓ red pepper flakes	✓ paprika	✓ saffron	
	✓ rosemary	✓ parsley	✓ star anise	
	✓ smoked paprika	✓ saffron	✓ thyme	

How to Read Food Labels

Another good reason to move toward a more whole plant-based diet is you won't be buying as many packaged foods—so there will be fewer labels to decipher (and less plastic waste). When you do, though, it helps if you know what you're looking at.

There are three things worth noting:

1. Don't be misled by the health claims on the package

I don't want to be a downer on your shopping experience or turn you into a skeptic, but those eye-grabbing health claims are often not what they seem. Take the many cereal boxes that shout "high fiber" and "immune support" on the front. When you turn them around and dig a little deeper, in more cases than not the fiber comes from a single refined powder, such as chicory root fiber (no plant diversity here!), and the added sugars are twice that of the fiber—not to mention the vast collection of food additives.

In terms of immune health, any product with a certain level of micronutrients, including vitamins C or B6, can claim that it supports your "immune health," despite the vast majority of us already getting more than enough of those vitamins from our diets. And yes, even those sugar-loaded breakfast cereals with token vitamins added in can make these claims.

2. All the secrets lie in the ingredient list

Forget what the product name is or what it might say on the front; the ingredient list tells you what's really in it. Ingredients are listed from greatest to smallest by weight. So that "blueberry" cereal bar you bought might have lots of other ingredients higher up the list than actual blueberries (which may be present in a tiny amount, or only as a dried extract or even artificial flavoring, meaning it may not even contain any blueberry at all!).

It's worth being an "added sugar" spy, too, because on ingredient lists it often hides in various different disguises: glucose, dextrose, fructose, maltose, sucrose, lactose, syrup (date, maple, corn, brown rice, oat), honey, maltodextrin, agave nectar, fruit juice . . . to name just a few. While, yes, a little added sugar is completely fine ("a little" generally means that sugar appears near the end of the ingredient list), don't let them sneak up on you in products disguised as "healthy."

3. Nutrition information is a comparison game, not about black-and-white rules

Next, you can look to the nutrition facts, which are usually displayed in a table, like the one on page 107, and details: fat (including saturated fat), protein, carbohydrates (including sugars, both naturally occurring and added), salt (often referenced as "sodium") and energy (measured in calories). Generally, it'll also list any vitamins and minerals, as well as fiber, if present in significant amounts. Labels will usually give you amounts for these according to serving size, as well as listing the number of servings contained in the overall package. But beware, this is one of the marketers' favorite tricks—shrinking down the serving size to unrealistically small portions, just to get the pesky calories or sugars down in the table.

As you know by now, I don't typically recommend counting calories or measuring macros like carbs or fat. But I do suggest you get label-savvy, so you can read between the lines and find the products that are best for you. Most often, the product with the highest fiber and least salt and sugars (especially if the ingredient list suggests these sugars are added and not from whole fruit) makes it into my shopping cart. In terms of fat and protein, it really depends on the source of these nutrients—e.g., if the fats are coming from whole seeds and nuts (and not refined oils such as palm oil), then in my shopping cart they go. Again, this is why you should pay the most attention to the ingredient list! If you're counting anything, count the number of plants, not calories.

Tip
Aim to buy items that have whole foods listed within the first three ingredients. Added sugars should be low on the list if it's a daily food item.

Fat: Remember, fat is not to be feared, and it's more about the source than the total fat amount. There is strong evidence that we should all be reducing trans fats, and artificial trans fats are banned in the US.

Sodium: Choose lower-sodium options among similar foods—you can use the % DV to help. Other names for higher-sodium ingredients: baking powder, celery salt, garlic salt, meat/yeast extract, monosodium glutamate (MSG), onion salt, sea salt, sodium, sodium ascorbate, sodium bicarbonate, sodium nitrate/nitrite, stock cubes, vegetable salt.

Total sugars and added sugars: This includes both naturally occurring (e.g., from whole fruit and dairy) and added sugars. Avoiding sugar isn't necessary, but try to limit larger amounts of added sugars. If sugar content per 100 g is more than 15 g, check that added sugar is not listed on the ingredients list. Other names for added sugar: glucose, dextrose, fructose, maltose, sucrose, lactose, syrup (date, maple, corn, brown rice), honey, maltodextrin, agave nectar, fruit juice.

Micronutrients: All labels must include vitamin D, calcium, iron, and potassium, because many people don't get enough of these. Including other micronutrients that may be present in a product, such as folate, is optional.

Nutrition Facts

4 servings per container
Serving size 1 1/2 cup (208g)

Amount per serving
Calories 240

	% Daily Value*
Total Fat 4g	**5%**
Saturated Fat 1.5g	**8%**
Trans Fat 0g	
Cholesterol 5mg	**2%**
Sodium 430mg	**19%**
Total Carbohydrate 46g	**17%**
Dietary fiber 7g	**25%**
Total Sugars 4g	
Includes 2g Added Sugars	**4%**
Protein 11g	
Vitamin D 2mcg	10%
Calcium 260mg	20%
Iron 6mg	35%
Potassium 240mg	6%

*The % Daily Value (DV) tells you how much a nutrient in a serving of food contributes to a daily diet. 2,000 calories a day is used for general nutrition advice.

INGREDIENTS: BULGUR WHEAT, SAUCE (WATER, HALF AND HALF [MILK, CREAM], PARMESAN CHEESE [PASTEURIZED SKIM MILK, CULTURES, SALT, ENZYMES], CHEDDAR CHEESE [PASTEURIZED MILK, CULTURES, SALT, ENZYMES], OLIVE OIL, BUTTER, SUGAR, XANTHAN GUM, SPICE), LENTILS, CORN, GREEN BEANS, RED BEANS, POTATOES.

Serving Size: This is not a health-based recommendation on how much to eat but rather an amount set by brands (often influenced by marketing strategies) to make a product look lower in calories or sugars than it really is. When comparing products, be sure to also check the serving sizes to ensure you're comparing like for like.

% Daily Value: A daily value (DV) is the amount of each nutrient recommended at a minimum (e.g., dietary fiber) or maximum (e.g., added sugars) each day. The percentage daily value therefore helps you to determine how much a nutrient in a serving of food contributes to your total daily diet. As a general guide, 5% DV or less of a nutrient per serving is considered low, and 20% DV or more of a nutrient per serving is considered high.

Fiber: Although the DV is set at 28 g, I recommend you try to aim above and beyond, as I discuss on page 16.

Ingredients: These are listed from greatest to smallest by weight. Use the list to check that at least the first three ingredients are whole foods. Remember, this is the section you should pay the most attention to.

Being Mindful about Eating

Paying a little attention to why and how we're eating goes a long way towards making healthier choices and having better gut health. Have you ever mindlessly eaten a package of cookies or a chocolate bar and found yourself, moments later, questioning where it went and second-guessing whether you really did eat the whole thing? Our busy lives have taught us that multitasking is an impressive skill, but this has led to so many of us eating mindlessly. The outcome? We feel less satisfied and are more likely to experience digestive issues. Highly processed foods in particular melt in our mouths (remember how little chewing they require!) so, particularly when we're distracted, we barely notice we're eating them. And therefore those satiety signals don't have time to register.

Fellow researchers have developed a questionnaire that I often use in my clinic to help clients reflect on their current eating habits, drivers and patterns. The questionnaire is on page 111, with downloadable copies available on theguthealthdoctor.com. Monitor your progress after implementing the ten-step mindful-eating exercise on page 110 for eight weeks.

Revamping your relationship with food

Eating mindfully means being aware, without judgment, of all the physical and emotional sensations of eating. It's a useful tool that can help build a healthier relationship with foods that may have previously been "banned" while dieting. If you're concerned that eating more plants will make you feel deprived, you feel out of control around some foods (peanut butter, I'm looking at you!), or you're struggling with cravings (remember, no food is off limits), I'd recommend making mindful eating part of your tool kit.

Supporting your digestion

If you're burdened by gut symptoms, such as bloating, mindful eating can be a real game-changer. By tuning into all your senses (sight, smell, feel, sound, and taste), your body becomes better prepared for the meal (enzymes are released, blood moves to your stomach, your "fight or flight" nervous system winds down and your "rest and digest" nervous system ramps up). In turn, your digestive system becomes more relaxed and can go about its job more efficiently.

Mindful-Eating Exercise

I'm certainly not expecting you to do this every time you eat—but I have a feeling once you give it a go and see the difference it makes to your eating experience, as many of my clients have, you may be inclined to do it more regularly.

The "eating with all your senses" exercise on page 110 is a really good one to try with a food you'd normally wolf down. A small bar of chocolate or a cookie, for example, or maybe your favorite meal. The ten-step exercise will walk you through this sensuous way of enjoying your food by savoring each mouthful; it's a great way to switch off guilt and gorging and turn on digestion.

If you're struggling with your relationship with certain foods, at a minimum I'd suggest you do this three times a week using a small portion of those foods. If digestive symptoms are more of your concern, try following the exercise for the first few mouthfuls of your main meal of the day. If you're able to keep doing the exercise regularly, you'll start to notice this mindful way of eating naturally becomes your new normal. For more food satisfaction, and less digestive distress, give it a go today!

Getting Ready

✓ Sit down at a table.

✓ Clear any clutter, make this just about your food.

✓ Set a place for yourself, even if it's just you, and make it look good—a nice glass, a napkin, the right lighting, some gentle music—it all counts.

✓ Take a few extra moments to present your food well. Put away your phone, tablet, magazine, the crossword—so you can focus on eating.

✓ Take a few deep breaths into your lower belly, close your eyes, and relax.

The Exercise: Ten Steps to Eating with All Your Senses

1. Appreciate the look of the food in front of you—the colors, shape, and form.

2. Close your eyes to engage more deeply with your other senses.

3. Notice the aroma of what you're about to eat. What does it remind you of? Can you smell different notes? Does your mouth start to water?

4. Take a forkful and your first taste by swiping your tongue over the food. How does it feel?

5. Take your first bite. How does it taste just sitting in your mouth?

6. As you start to chew, be aware of the textures and how they change.

7. Tune into the sounds—is the food bubbling? Fizzing? Is there a loud crunch when you bite into it? Try blocking your ears with your fingers to engage more deeply with the sound of each chew.

8. Focus on the taste. Does it change as the food moves around your mouth and the more you chew?

9. Notice how many times you tend to chew the food before you swallow. Consider its onward journey—can you feel it sliding down? Is there a taste left in your mouth?

10. How does eating this food make you feel? Are you enjoying it?

Being Mindful about Eating

The questions in this assessment look at both your awareness of how food **affects your senses** and your **ability to recognize when you're hungry and full.**

	Rarely/ Never	Sometimes	Often	Usually/ Always
Before I eat, I take a moment to appreciate colors and smells of food.	0	1	2	3
I notice when the food I eat affects my emotional state.	0	1	2	3
I taste every bite of food I eat.	0	1	2	3
When eating a pleasant meal, I notice if it makes me feel relaxed.	0	1	2	3
I appreciate the way my food looks on my plate.	0	1	2	3
I notice subtle flavors in the foods I eat.	0	1	2	3
I recognize when I am eating and not hungry.	0	1	2	3
I notice when foods and drinks are too sweet.	0	1	2	3
I recognize when food advertisements make me want to eat.	0	1	2	3
When I eat a big meal, I notice if it makes me feel heavy or sluggish.	0	1	2	3
I notice when I am eating from a dish of candy just because it's there.	0	1	2	3
If there is good food at a party, I will continue eating even after I'm full.	3	2	1	0
If there are leftovers that I like, I take a second helping even if I'm full.	3	2	1	0
When I eat at all-you-can-eat buffets, I tend to overeat.	3	2	1	0
I stop eating when I'm full even when eating something I love.	0	1	2	3
When a restaurant portion is too large, I stop eating when I'm full.	0	1	2	3
When I'm eating one of my favorite foods, I don't recognize when I've had enough.	3	2	1	0
At a party with a lot of good food, I notice when it makes me want to eat more than I should.	0	1	2	3
If it doesn't cost much more, I get the larger size food or drink regardless of how hungry I feel.	3	2	1	0
I snack without noticing that I'm eating.	3	2	1	0

Tally your score: _____

Score Interpretation

Let's bring some mindfulness to mealtimes.

Top marks! You've mastered mindful eating.

0 ⟶ 60

If your score is towards the lower end, rest assured you're not alone!

Dieting culture and our multitasking ways have influenced how many of us eat. Practicing mindful techniques, including the exercise on page 110, is a great place to start. After implementing the exercise at least 3 times per week for eight weeks, repeat the questionnaire so that you can monitor your progress.

Six Tips for Adapting to a Higher-Fiber Diet

We touched on how changing your diet to include more plants might affect those with sensitive guts in chapter 5, but I think all of us would benefit from a little awareness and preparation when it comes to upping our plant portions. Think of it like this: As your diet moves from a little to a lot of fiber, it's naturally going to provide quite the feast for your gut microbes. There may be some excitement, some fizzing and popping—aka that feeling of bloating and gassiness—as your microbes celebrate this new way of eating. But it certainly doesn't have to be that way. If you want to avoid too much gut "excitement," here are my top tips and tricks to building your tolerance (and your microbes' digestive capacity).

1. Go slow and build up gradually.

Don't transform your diet overnight or binge on plants one day and deprive your microbes the next. Like us, they need "food" every day to function at their best. If you're worried about how to do this, my menu plan for Sensitive Guts (see pages 124 to 125) will help guide you.

2. Stay hydrated.

Fiber needs water to "perform" at its best. So, as you up your fiber, remember to up your water, too.

3. Chew your food well.

When it comes to high-fiber whole foods, aim to chew each mouthful around twenty times. This not only helps prep your stomach for the incoming food, but it also kickstarts the digestive process that occurs in your mouth (both physically with your teeth and chemically with the enzymes in your saliva).

4. Keep moving.

Staying active doesn't support just your arm and leg muscles, but your digestive muscles, too (remember your digestive tract is wrapped in muscle!).

5. Stretch it out.

Feeling bloated? Some gentle yoga-like stretching at the end of the day (when, typically, symptoms are at their peak after a day full of food) can help. Try cat-cow, happy baby, and crocodile twist, before resting in child's pose for five deep belly breaths (I demonstrate all of these postures in *Love Your Gut*).

6. Worship the heat pack.

For those of you who do experience a little extra gut activity, remember that it's nothing to be worried about. But if it's uncomfortable, applying a heat pack to your stomach can work wonders by drawing extra blood there to support digestion.

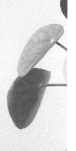

De-Stressing the Gut

Good gut health doesn't entirely come down to diet. There are other factors that can adversely affect your gut health, in particular stress and poor sleep—as those of you with sensitive guts probably know only too well.

A little bit of stress is healthy. Without it, we'd never study for an exam, hit a personal best, or achieve many of our goals. But, like all things, there's a fine balance between helpful stress and stress as a hindrance. Whether it's the influx of stress hormones like cortisol playing havoc with our digestive systems, or the angry messages shooting down the communication highway between our brain and gut, chronic stress is a common barrier to good gut health.

A lack of quality sleep is another barrier many of my clients face. Sleep is vital for rest and regeneration, and that goes for your gut, too. Indeed, parts of your gut lining shed and regenerate every week or so, and it needs you to be well rested for this to happen efficiently. Studies have also shown that after just two days of sleep deprivation, your GM is negatively impacted. This is because, like us, our gut microbes have a circadian rhythm (sleep–wake cycle), and if we disturb ours, we disturb theirs, too.

Thankfully, there are now plenty of research-backed strategies to help us all combat the inevitable periods of stress and poor sleep that modern life throws at us. Check out my seven favorite exercises on pages 114 to 115—they really can make a difference to how you feel.

How to De-Stress and Sleep Better

I know "reduce stress and sleep better" is hardly useful advice in practice. If it were that easy, I wouldn't be writing this section. So, instead, here's my handy list of evidence-based suggestions that have really worked for my clients.

1. Dose up on the cuddle hormone.

Whether it's a hug from someone else or one from yourself, the physical sensation of touch has been shown to activate nerves that, in turn, trigger the increase of oxytocin, the "cuddle hormone." This release provides a sense of safety, soothes any feelings of distress, and calms that "fight or flight" sympathetic nervous system. Give it a try, really focusing on how you feel with the initial contact and holding.

2. Treat self-care as a necessity, not a luxury.

Whether you're tending to your kids' every need, working crazy hours, or busy being a good friend . . . you don't just deserve some dedicated "me-time"—you need it, or you will absolutely burn out. Whether it's taking a candlelit bubble bath or treating yourself to a solo coffee date, scheduling at least a few thirty-minute self-care sessions each week is well worth the time investment.

3. Acknowledge and accept your feelings.

Here's one of my favorite quotes, from poet Nayyirah Waheed: "and I said to my body softly, 'I want to be your friend.' It took a long breath and replied, 'I have been waiting my whole life for this.'" Sometimes we run the risk of ignoring or even suppressing our thoughts and feelings. In fact, in my clinic I often find gut issues are worse in those whose stress is subconscious. Being able to suppress emotions may be a nifty skill for combating acute stress, but in the long term these emotions often scream out via your gut. How are you feeling right now? Deep down? Acknowledge it's okay to feel that way. Say to yourself out loud, "I am feeling . . . and it's okay to feel that way."

4. Keep a gratitude diary.

At the end of each day, list three things that happened that you're grateful for. It could be a smile from a stranger, a call from a friend, or a nice email from a colleague. As simple as it sounds, reflecting on the good things can "rewire" how your brain thinks over time, creating more inner peace and calm—no matter your external environment.

5. Do a five-minute body scan.

In a relaxed, seated position, with your eyes closed, imagine a gentle flow of warm liquid light trickling down from above your head through your body, filling up gradually from your pinky toes. Notice the liquid's calming quality filling up your feet, through your ankles, into your lower legs . . . Continue for several minutes to visualize it filling each individual part of your body until it reaches the top of your head. Let it overflow, covering your skin with a warming touch. Slowly open your eyes and reflect on how you feel.

6. Try box breathing.

Breathe in through your nose for four seconds, hold for four, exhale slowly and steadily through your nose for four, hold for four. Repeat for ten cycles. The holding of breath changes the amount of carbon dioxide in the body, which through a sequence of mechanisms activates your "rest and digest" nervous system, aka your parasympathetic system. The result? A wave of calm moves through your body. Try it!

7. Go forest bathing.

This is just another term for mindfully spending time in nature. Rain, hail, or shine, develop curiosity for how your body feels as you walk through nature, as each foot lands on the ground. It's all about being present with those otherwise automatic and unconscious movements. And while "being with nature" may sound a bit hippie-dippie, a body of research, including fourteen studies, has shown that forest bathing really does lower stress levels and even high blood pressure.

Getting Started on Your Journey

It's really up to you how you approach the Diversity Diet. You may want to embrace all the tips in this chapter and dive into my recipes, or perhaps you'd prefer just to dip your toe in and start by tracking your weekly plant points (see page 27) for a more gradual approach. Whether you start by focusing on one meal a day—breakfast, lunch, or dinner—or just try some of my one-minute snack ideas (see pages 304 to 305), as long as you're moving in the direction of plant-based diversity, your microbes will absolutely appreciate your efforts.

My approach to food is very practical. The recipes are for you to use every day, and you don't need to be a skilled cook to make any of them (I'm certainly not!). You'll notice a range of features, indicated with icons at the top of the page, including **freezer-suitable** recipes, perfect for batch-cooking ahead of time for busy weeks; recipes that can be made **FODMAP-lite** for people with more sensitive guts (see pages 306 to 310 for detailed switches for each recipe); **Fridge Raids**, where you use up any fruit and veggies that are about to go bad, and **zero-waste** recipes, so you can do your bit for saving the planet (and save money, too!). There are also a few "reinvented" recipes, where you can use the leftovers from a dinner recipe to create a tasty lunch the next day (pages 207, 209, and 210). My hope is that after seeing how easy and delicious this way of eating is for yourself, you'll consider cooking for friends and family, too—and together discover some of the incredible tastes, textures, and experiences that come with embracing the Diversity Diet.

 Freezer   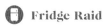 FODMAP-Lite   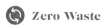 Fridge Raid   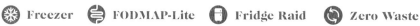 Zero Waste

I know from experience with clients—and from your messages about *Love Your Gut*—that lots of you love a little more guidance to help you change your habits. So I've created three different menu plans for different lifestyles: Fueling Families, Busy People, and Sensitive Guts. Pick one or try all three. My hope is that these menu plans act as a blueprint for you to adapt, based on the recipes that work best for you, your microbes, and your lifestyle. Let's take a closer look . . .

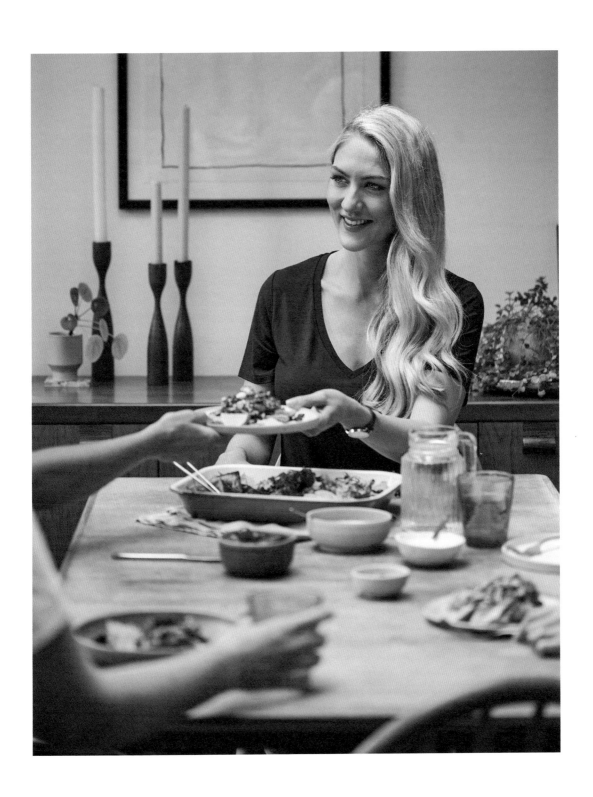

The Diversity Diet Menu Plans

Plan 1 is for FUELING FAMILIES

My most versatile plan, with child-friendly meals and fun ideas. Be sure to check serving sizes to suit your family's needs.

Plan 2 is for BUSY PEOPLE

None of the suggested weekday recipes in this plan take longer than twenty minutes to whip up, and many are ready in just five.

Plan 3 is for SENSITIVE GUTS

This plan features FODMAP-lite options (see pages 306 to 310 for more on this), so you can banish all that plant-based prejudice that often comes with a sensitive gut and start to reap the benefits.

For each plan, I've picked out recipes from the book to give you a whole week's kick-start menu. Each one delivers at least 30 different plant points, along with gut-loving prebiotics, phytochemicals, and over 30 grams of fiber per day. In fact, if you follow the plans to a T, including snacks and desserts, you'll be getting close to 80 plant points across the week and 50 grams of fiber each day! And you'll be happy to know this doesn't mean extra time, complexity, or cost on your part. It's all thanks to simple hacks covered on pages 94 and 95. As you get to know the recipes and what works for you, you can start to build your own menu plan—you can find a printable copy on my website (theguthealthdoctor.com).

I've tried and tested each of these menu plans and found that prepping a few recipes on the weekend makes a world of difference for the week ahead, so in each plan I've flagged a few of the recipes that are worth making in advance. I've designed them to fit around your life and not vice versa, but feel free to mix and match or even batch-cook your favorite recipes. I hope they help to steer you as you get going.

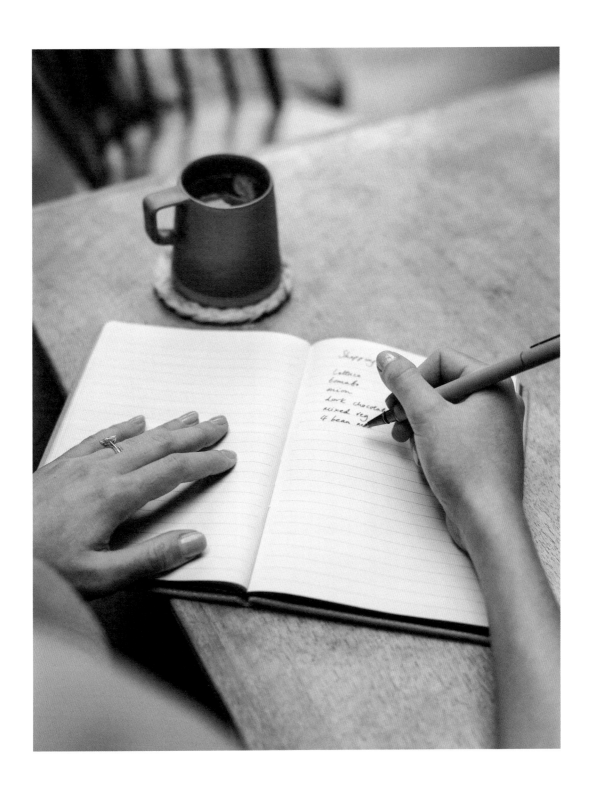

Fueling Families

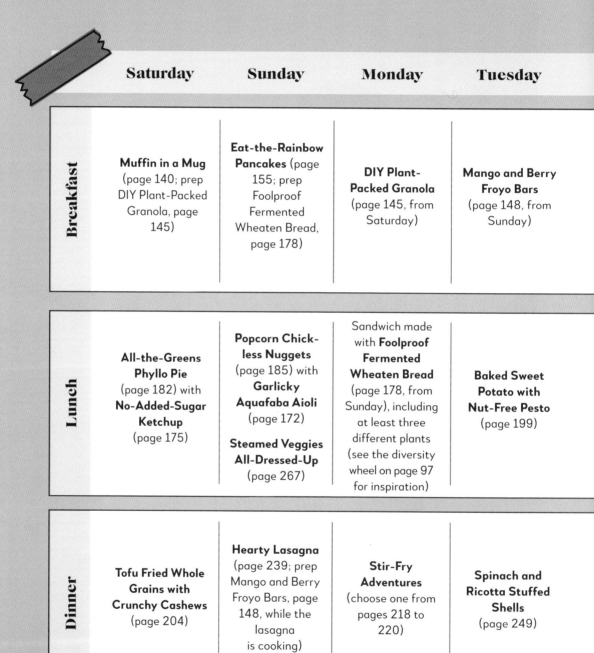

	Saturday	Sunday	Monday	Tuesday
Breakfast	**Muffin in a Mug** (page 140; prep DIY Plant-Packed Granola, page 145)	**Eat-the-Rainbow Pancakes** (page 155; prep Foolproof Fermented Wheaten Bread, page 178)	**DIY Plant-Packed Granola** (page 145, from Saturday)	**Mango and Berry Froyo Bars** (page 148, from Sunday)
Lunch	**All-the-Greens Phyllo Pie** (page 182) with **No-Added-Sugar Ketchup** (page 175)	**Popcorn Chick-less Nuggets** (page 185) with **Garlicky Aquafaba Aioli** (page 172) **Steamed Veggies All-Dressed-Up** (page 267)	Sandwich made with **Foolproof Fermented Wheaten Bread** (page 178, from Sunday), including at least three different plants (see the diversity wheel on page 97 for inspiration)	**Baked Sweet Potato with Nut-Free Pesto** (page 199)
Dinner	**Tofu Fried Whole Grains with Crunchy Cashews** (page 204)	**Hearty Lasagna** (page 239; prep Mango and Berry Froyo Bars, page 148, while the lasagna is cooking)	**Stir-Fry Adventures** (choose one from pages 218 to 220)	**Spinach and Ricotta Stuffed Shells** (page 249)

Wednesday	Thursday	Friday
DIY Plant-Packed Granola (page 145, from Saturday)	**No-Bake Fruit and Nut Bites** (page 144)	**DIY Plant-Packed Granola** (page 145, from Saturday)
Snack-o-Clock Veggie Fritters (page 181) with **Garlicky Aquafaba Aioli** (page 172, from Sunday)	**Green Pea and "Ham" Soup** (page 232) with **Foolproof Fermented Wheaten Bread** (page 178, from Sunday)	**Reinvented Chicken Burger** (page 207, using 1 batch leftover Chicken 'n' Veggie Meatball mix from Thursday) with **No-Added-Sugar Ketchup** (page 175, from Saturday)
Creamy Dairy-Free Linguine (page 227)	**Chicken 'n' Veggie Meatballs** (page 258, make a double batch) **Fried Quinoa with Hoisin Drizzle** (page 273)	**Loaded Vegan Nachos** (page 233)

Snacks & Desserts

- **Loaded Melon Wedges** (page 159)
- **Seedy Cracker Duo** (page 177)
- **Cream-less Ice Cream** (page 279, prep the day before)
- **Fruit and Nut Wheels** (page 160)
- **Prebiotic Cookie Dough Drops** (page 165)
- **Chocolate Chip Zucchini Cookies** (page 291)
- **Raspberry Red Smoothie** (page 297)
- **Prebiotic Rocky Road** (page 283)
- **Snickers Smoothie Bowl** (page 295)

One-Minute Snacks

- **Banana Bites** (page 304)
- **Beans 'n' Crackers** (page 305, use any leftover cashew cheese from Friday's Loaded Vegan Nachos)
- **Prebiotic "Chocolate" Milkshake** (page 304)
- **Apple Slider** (page 304)
- **Sweet Potato Slider** (page 304, using leftover Baked Sweet Potato from Tuesday)

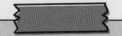

Busy People

	Saturday	Sunday	Monday	Tuesday
Breakfast	Breakfast Pita Pizza (page 153)	Plant-Powered Baked Oat Bars (page 150) or No-Bake Fruit and Nut Bites (page 144)	Immunity-Nourishing Smoothie (page 296)	Omelet Bowl (page 141) Frothy Cashew Latte (page 302)
Lunch	Thai-Inspired Fish Cakes and Crunchy Salad (page 212)	Phyllo Parcels with Saucy Mushrooms (page 224)	Leafy Taco Wraps (page 187)	Butternut Muffins (page 191, from Sunday)
Dinner	Tear-and-Share Bread with Butter Bean Relish (page 250) Steamed Veggies All Dressed Up (page 267, optional side)	Butternut Muffins (page 191)	Reinvented Saucy Mushroom Pita Pockets (page 209, using leftover mushrooms from Sunday's Phyllo Parcels)	Stir-Fry Adventures (choose one from pages 218 to 220)

Wednesday	Thursday	Friday
Plant-Powered Baked Oat Bars (page 150) or **No-Bake Fruit and Nut Bites** (page 144, leftover from Sunday)	**Fiber-Filled Breakfast Wrap** (page 143)	**Muffin in a Mug** (page 140) **Frothy Cashew Latte** (page 302)
Baked Sweet Potato with Black Beans (page 198)	**Zucchini and Hazelnut Salad** (page 186)	**Beet, Lentil, and Goat Cheese Salad** (page 195)
Green Pea and "Ham" Soup (page 232)	**Stir-Fry Adventures** (choose one from pages 218 to 220)	**Easy Noodle Soup** (page 231)

Snacks & Desserts

- **Trail Mix Loaf Cake with Yogurt and White Chocolate Glaze** (page 278, skip the glaze to store in the freezer)
- **Stuffed Dates, Four Ways** (page 167)
- **Cream-less Ice Cream** (page 279, no-freeze option)
- **Four-Ingredient Citrus Bars** (page 169)

One-Minute Snacks

- **Sweet Potato Slider** (page 304, using leftover Baked Sweet Potato from Wednesday)
- **Zucchini Slider** (page 305, using leftover tomato base from Saturday's Breakfast Pita Pizza as the dip)
- **Prebiotic "Chocolate" Milkshake** (page 304)
- **Froyo Berries** (page 305)
- **Mediterranean Stack** (page 305)
- **Apple Slider** (page 304)
- **Banana Bites** (page 304)
- **Bean Dippers** (page 304)
- **Avo Slider** (page 305)
- **Beans 'N' Crackers** (page 305)

Don't have a minute? Try: fresh fruit, one 5.3 ounce (150 g) container of probiotic yogurt, a handful of mixed nuts, or hummus with a whole carrot or a celery stick instead.

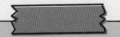

Sensitive Guts

	Saturday	Sunday	Monday	Tuesday
Breakfast	Crispy Bacon-Shrooms with Creamy Butter Bean Hummus (page 146)	Plant-Powered Baked Oat Bars (page 150) Frothy Cashew Latte (page 302)	Fiber-Filled Breakfast Wrap (page 143)	Omelet Bowl (page 141)
Lunch	Chunky Veggie and Feta Frittata (page 203)	Butternut Muffins (page 191)	Chunky Veggie and Feta Frittata (page 203, from Saturday)	Baked Sweet Potato with Nut-Free Pesto (page 199)
Dinner	Orange-Glazed Roasted Salmon (page 228) and Sticky Parsnips (page 266)	All-the-Greens Phyllo Pie (page 182) with **Garlicky Aquafaba Aioli** (page 172)	Stir-Fry Adventures (choose one from pages 218 to 220)	Chicken 'n' Veggie Meatballs (page 258) with **Fried Quinoa with Hoisin Drizzle** (page 273)

Wednesday	Thursday	Friday
Immunity-Nourishing Smoothie (page 296)	Plant-Powered Baked Oat Bars (page 150, from Sunday)	Muffin in a Mug (page 140) Frothy Cashew Latte (page 302)
Reinvented Chicken Burgers (page 207, using leftover chicken meatball mixture)	Zucchini and Hazelnut Salad (page 186)	Butternut Muffins (page 191, from Sunday)
Thai-Inspired Fish Cakes and Crunchy Salad (page 212)	Popcorn Chick-less Nuggets (page 185) with Garlicky Aquafaba Aioli (page 172, from Sunday) Steamed Veggies All Dressed Up (page 267)	Stir-Fry Adventures (choose one from pages 218 to 220)

Snacks & Desserts

- **Chocolate Chip Zucchini Cookies** (page 291)
- **Ultimate Raspberry and White Chocolate Muffins** (page 163)
- **Trail Mix Loaf Cake with Yogurt and White Chocolate Glaze** (page 278)
- **Seedy Cracker Duo** (page 177) with leftover **Creamy Butter Bean Hummus** (page 146, from Saturday) and tomato
- **Cream-less Ice Cream** (page 280, no-freeze option)
- **Pistachio Berry Bursts** (page 284)
- **Raspberry and Lemon Ricotta Cheesecake** (page 277)
- **Spinach Balls with Tahini Sauce** (page 270)

One-Minute Snacks

- **Mediterranean Stack** (page 305)
- **Zucchini Slider** (page 305, using leftover butter bean hummus from Saturday's Crispy Bacon-Shrooms as the dip)
- **Banana Bites** (page 304)
- **Bean Dippers** (page 304)
- **Avo Slider** (page 305)
- **Prebiotic "Chocolate" Milkshake** (page 304)

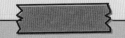

See the FODMAP-lite tweaks and portion guidance, which are detailed for each recipe at the back of the book on pages 306 to 310.

FODMAP-Lite Foods

If you've read my first book, chances are you'll know quite a lot about FODMAPs. But if not, here's a quick recap of the basics and how they tie into the Sensitive Guts menu plan.

FODMAP is an acronym for a group of carbohydrates, many of which are prebiotic fibers that your gut microbes love to eat. However, for those with more sensitive guts, loading up on too many FODMAPs at once may trigger gut symptoms, such as uncomfortable bloating, extra gas, altered poops, and more. The low-FODMAP diet is a medical diet that involves a restriction stage that cuts out all high-FODMAP foods. The restriction stage eliminates certain foods—including garlic, onions, apples, and most legumes—that are ordinarily loved by your GM. This has been shown to be effective in providing short-term relief, particularly in people with severe irritable bowel syndrome (IBS).

But there are several risks attached to the strict nature of the diet—if this restriction phase is followed for more than eight weeks, you risk starving off and unbalancing your GM long-term. In fact, research has shown that extended restriction leads to a reduction in beneficial microbes such as *Bifidobacteria*, the very bacteria that have been linked to a decrease in some IBS symptoms. Go figure! So instead, I've developed a much less intensive and lower-risk approach, which I call FODMAP-lite. My approach reduces the FODMAP load, giving sensitive guts more time to adapt without cutting these gut-loving foods out completely.

The recipes with the ⊜ icon can be made FODMAP-lite by making switches and watching the portions outlined for each recipe on pages 306 to 310. The FODMAP-lite recipes don't restrict lactose—i.e., milk sugar—so if you know lactose is an issue for you, substitute lactose-free yogurt or milk. I've also included a list of general FODMAP switches on page 311.

The most common FODMAP-lite switches:

Dates/date paste ➡ maple syrup

Garlic ➡ garlic-infused olive oil

Onion ➡ chives or the green parts of scallions

Wheat, spelt, or rye flour and whole grains ➡ gluten-free flour and whole grains

---

Soy or oat milk ➡ almond milk

Legumes ➡ canned legumes, triple-rinsed with water (stick to ¼ cup/45 g per serving)

If high-FODMAP foods are a concern for you, be sure to check out the full FODMAP-lite guide in my first book, *Love Your Gut*. This includes more information about the reintroduction and personalization stages of the FODMAP-lite approach, which are key to nourishing your gut in the long term.

Plant Points Planner

Whether you're following the menu plans or not, I've created this planner for you to keep track of the plant points you eat each week (there's a blank one on my website for you to print off, too). The aim is to record the plants you've eaten each day, then tally up your points (turn to page 27 for a reminder of what counts toward your total). Remember that you only record each ingredient once a week, so don't worry if you're just scoring one or two a day by the end of the week—that's normal, especially if you batch-cook—it's the

	Saturday	Sunday	Monday	Tuesday
Date:	6/25	6/26		
Week 1	**Whole grains:** Oats, wheat berries	**Whole grains:** Quinoa	**Whole grains:**	**Whole grains:**
	Fruit: Dates, red apple, mango	**Fruit:** Strawberries, blueberries	**Fruit:**	**Fruit:**
	Vegetables: Beets, onion, watercress, carrot, celery, red cabbage	**Vegetables:** Portobello mushrooms, butternut squash, zucchini, corn	**Vegetables:**	**Vegetables:**
	Nuts & seeds: Almonds, sunflower and pumpkin seeds	**Nuts & seeds:** Walnuts, chia seeds	**Nuts & seeds:**	**Nuts & seeds:**
	Legumes: Chickpeas, butter beans	**Legumes:** Soy beans	**Legumes:**	**Legumes:**
	Herbs & spices: Coffee, basil, paprika, EVOO	**Herbs & spices:** Garlic, cocoa, cinnamon	**Herbs & spices:**	**Herbs & spices:**
	Daily Total: Plant Points 17	**Daily Total:** Plant Points 10.75	**Daily Total:** Plant Points	**Daily Total:** Plant Points

weekly total that counts, and if you've got more than 30, your gut microbes will be thrilled! On each of my recipes, I've included how many plant points they provide if you follow them to a T, but make sure to record what you actually ate. For example, if you used mixed seeds rather than just sunflower seeds, remember to count each variety. It all adds up—the more the merrier!

Wednesday	Thursday	Friday
Whole grains:	Whole grains:	Whole grains:
Fruit:	Fruit:	Fruit:
Vegetables:	Vegetables:	Vegetables:
Nuts & seeds:	Nuts & seeds:	Nuts & seeds:
Legumes:	Legumes:	Legumes:
Herbs & spices:	Herbs & spices:	Herbs & spices:
Daily Total: *Plant Points*	Daily Total: *Plant Points*	Daily Total: *Plant Points*

Weekly Total:

Plant Points

The 28-Day Plant Points Challenge

Are you up for a gut health challenge? I've put together this plant-packed 28-day challenge to make it even easier for you to up your plant points, reaching 30 plants and beyond each week.

It's as simple as completing one challenge (set out on page 132) per day for 28 days. If you want to go that extra mile, keep a tally of your plant points each week (see page 128 for your template) and try to beat your plant points score each week.

Why not get a friend, family member or work colleague on board? The more the merrier! Share your journey on social media with #plantpointschallenge. I'd love to follow!

Once you experience the benefit for yourself, I've got a feeling you'll want to continue beyond the 28 days, which is where the menu plans on page 133 can come in!

How Healthy Is Your Gut?

Before you begin the challenge, for those who love objective "data," I recommend you complete this assessment so that you can see how this challenge might benefit you. After the 28-day challenge, answer these questions again to see which areas have improved. For each question, select the answer that applies to you, then add up your score.

1. How often are you bothered by gut symptoms (e.g., bloating, reflux, constipation)?

Less than once per month	1 to 3 times per month	1 to 2 times per week	3 or more times per month
(3 points)	*(2 points)*	*(1 point)*	*(0 points)*

2. Do you take regular medication or over-the-counter drugs (including the contraceptive pill)?

No	Yes
(2 points)	*(0 points)*

3. Do any health conditions run in your family (e.g. diabetes, high blood pressure)?

No	Yes
(2 points)	*(0 points)*

4. How many different plant-based foods do you eat each week? (Including whole grains, legumes, vegetables, fruits, nuts, and seeds; herbs and spices count as a quarter of a point).

Fewer than 10	10 to 19	20 to 29	30+
(0 points)	*(1 point)*	*(2 points)*	*(3 points)*

5. In an average week, how would you describe yourself?

Unhappy	Neutral	Happy
(0 points)	*(1 point)*	*(2 points)*

6. How often are you unwell (e.g., with colds and flu)?

Not in the past month	Once in the past month	More than once per month
(2 points)	*(1 point)*	*(0 points)*

7. Are you avoiding any foods because of a suspected or diagnosed food intolerance?

No	Yes
(2 points)	*(0 points)*

8. How many hours do you sleep per night on average?

5 hours or fewer	More than 5 hours and less than 7	At least 7 hours
(0 points)	*(1 point)*	*(2 points)*

9. How often are you negatively impacted by stress?

Not in the past month	1 to 3 times in the past month	Every week
(2 points)	*(1 point)*	*(0 points)*

10. How often do you exercise (for at least 30 minutes) to a level where you'd become short of breath if you tried to sing?

Less than once per week	1 to 2 times per week	3 or more times per week
(0 points)	*(1 point)*	*(2 points)*

Tally your score: _____

0 points ⟶	20 points
Let's get to work!	Great job!

Your Plant Points Challenge

Here are your challenges for the next 28 days . . .

CHALLENGE 1

Try 1 to 2 fresh or frozen fruits you've never had before

CHALLENGE 2

Grate carrot, zucchini (or both!) into your breakfast oats or omelet

CHALLENGE 3

Enjoy a nutty dip (like Creamy Pistachio Dip, page 173)

CHALLENGE 4

Add an extra ½ cup of mixed frozen (or fresh) veggies to your dinner

CHALLENGE 5

Fill a jar with mixed seeds & sprinkle onto at least one meal today

CHALLENGE 6

Blend a new vegetable (e.g., spinach, carrot, frozen cauliflower, or cucumber) into your smoothie

CHALLENGE 7

Make chips using veggie peels (drizzle with olive oil and bake at 350°F/180°C for 15 to 25 minutes until crisp)

CHALLENGE 8

Experiment with a new whole grain (see pages 100–1 for inspiration)

CHALLENGE 9

Try a side of fermented food (e.g., kimchi or sauerkraut) with lunch or dinner

CHALLENGE 10

Have a prebiotic snack, like Seed 'n' Nut Stuffed Dates (page 167)

CHALLENGE 11

Go for veggie sticks and hummus as your afternoon snack (see Creamy Butter Bean Hummus, page 146)

CHALLENGE 12

Add an extra veggie topping (slices of tomato, mushroom, or greens) to your pizza

CHALLENGE 13

Cook up some plant protein (e.g., legumes or tofu; see Popcorn Chickless Nuggets, page 185)

CHALLENGE 14

Enjoy a polyphenol-packed snack (e.g., olives and avocado on whole grain crackers)

CHALLENGE 15

Add roasted veggies (e.g., peppers, eggplant, red onion) to a sandwich

CHALLENGE 16

Swap out white (pasta, rice, bread) for whole grain

CHALLENGE 17

Enjoy a quick 10 minute stir-fry with pre-cut veggies (see Stir-Fry Adventures, pages 218–20)

CHALLENGE 18

Blend some beans into your soup (see Green Pea and "Ham" Soup, page 232)

CHALLENGE 19

Quick snack: an apple, nut butter & mixed seeds

CHALLENGE 20

Add a mixed side salad to your takeout

CHALLENGE 21

Prep 2 different types of veggie sticks for the week ahead (e.g., green beans, sugar snap peas, or asparagus)

CHALLENGE 22

Use up any leftover veggies in your fridge in a wrap (see Fiber-Filled Breakfast Wrap, page 143)

CHALLENGE 23

Switch your single piece of fruit for ½ cup of mixed berries (fresh or frozen)

CHALLENGE 24

Curb those cravings with dark chocolate & mixed nuts (see Prebiotic Rocky Road, page 283)

CHALLENGE 25

Add a new canned legume to your dinner (e.g., black beans or lentils with pasta, pizza, or curry)

CHALLENGE 26

Add fresh herbs to your lunch (e.g., basil, cilantro, or parsley)

CHALLENGE 27

Befriend jarred veggies: Add beets, capers, or roasted peppers to your lunch

CHALLENGE 28

Add a handful of baby spinach or greens in the last 2 minutes of making a soup, stir-fry, or stew

Enjoy a mocktail (see Microbe-Made Ginger Soda, pages 300–1) to celebrate—challenge complete!

Easy Meal Ideas

Hitting your 30 plant points each week doesn't need to be complicated. It's about small tweaks and additions to your regular meals that make all the difference.

Here are some quick and simple meal ideas you can try—no recipe required.

	BREAKFAST	LUNCH	DINNER	SNACKS & SWEETS
MONDAY	Oatmeal topped with banana & mixed berries	Whole wheat wrap, mixed greens, cucumber, asparagus, hummus, & seeds	Mixed roasted veggies (sweet potato, onions, zucchini) with quinoa & pesto	Whole wheat crackers with avocado, tomatoes & fresh basil
TUESDAY	Mixed beans & beets on whole wheat seeded toast	Baked potato, mixed beans, cabbage, & parmesan/nutritional yeast	Whole wheat pasta with chopped tomatoes/passata & canned lentils	Crudités (green beans, cucumber, carrot) with hummus
WEDNESDAY	Smoothie with spinach, frozen fruit, oats & probiotic yogurt	Veggie omelet: eggs, peas, spinach, mushrooms, peppers & feta	Stir-fry with premixed veggies, soba noodles & soy sauce	Roasted chickpeas sprinkled with ground cumin, cilantro & paprika
THURSDAY	Eggs on sourdough, roasted tomatoes, leeks & mixed greens	Mix & match bowl: brown rice, mixed veggies, pumpkin seeds, tofu & soy sauce	Pita pizza with tomato puree, mushrooms, spinach & feta	Dark chocolate & mixed nuts
FRIDAY	Overnight oats soaked in milk of choice with apple & mixed seeds	Stuffed pita with falafel, probiotic yogurt, mixed greens & beets	Sheet pan meal: salmon, potatoes, green beans, cherry tomatoes & olives	Berry ice cream: blended frozen berries, banana & probiotic yogurt
SATURDAY	Probiotic yogurt with grated carrot, mixed berries & nuts	Butter beans, cashews & tomato salad topped with mango & avocado	Sourdough with hummus, roasted peppers, kale & mixed seeds	Medjool dates stuffed with tahini & sprinkled with mixed nuts
SUNDAY	Mixed mushrooms on whole grain seeded bread	Sweet potato, tomatoes, olives, mixed greens, olive oil & lemon juice	Grilled eggplant, zucchini & cauliflower with quinoa	Pear slices topped with probiotic yogurt, berries & chopped nuts

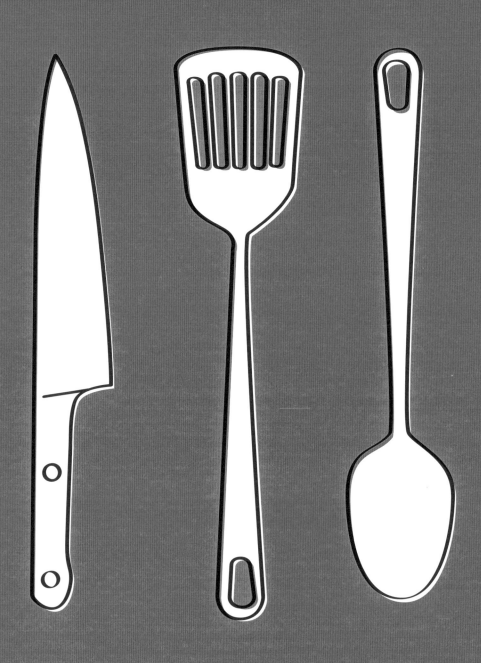

Part 2: Recipes

A Note on Ingredients

Peeling

Where I haven't specified peeling your plants, keep the skins on (just rinse well). This will not only save you time, but give you extra fiber, too.

Oil

Did you know that it's safe to cook with good-quality extra virgin olive oil (EVOO)? Research has shown it may be even more stable in home cooking (up to 450°F, 240°C for 20 minutes) than other oils, including sunflower, canola, and coconut oil. That's thanks to its high plant-chemical content and its antioxidant powers, which protect the fat from breaking down. Given the wealth of health benefits attributed to EVOO, it's what I recommend using in most of my recipes. (However, feel free to switch it out for your oil/fat of choice—it's your call.)

How do you spot "good quality" EVOO? Check: (1) The label includes both a best before and a harvest date; (2) The oil is stored in a dark glass bottle; and (3) The bottle has a certified stamp on it.

Nuts and seeds

Not that into them? Roasting them in the oven or frying pan for two minutes (even if I haven't specified it in the recipe) really does transform their taste and aroma and gives them that all-important crunch. While it may slightly change the nutritional properties, in the grand scheme of your diet it's rather negligible, especially if the alternative is skipping them altogether.

Sweeteners

Unlike added sugars (see page 107 for a list) whole dates are loaded with both gut-loving prebiotics and phytochemicals, such as flavonoids. This is why I tend to use whole Medjool dates as my sweetener of choice in these recipes. Simply use the back of a spoon to mash down one pitted date with 2 tablespoons of hot water until it forms a paste. Where the recipe calls for 2 dates, increase the water to ¼ cup (60 ml), and so on. If dates aren't your thing, feel free to swap in your sweetener of choice, such as maple syrup or honey (1 date = 1 tablespoon of sweetener = 15 grams).

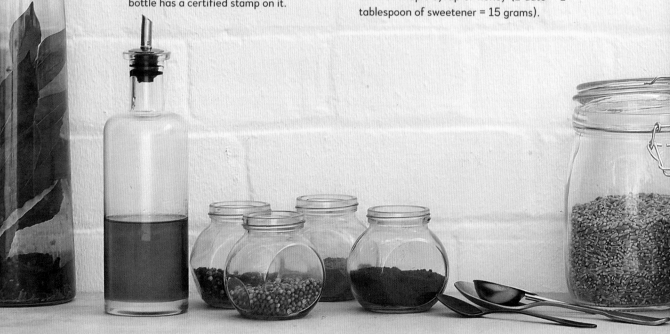

Measurements

Unless specified, ingredient weights are given as prepped weight.

Probiotic yogurt

Although all yogurt requires live bacteria to produce, a lot of these probiotic bacteria can die before they make it into your shopping cart. For reassurance that you're getting a decent amount of live bacteria, I recommend opting for yogurts that declare "probiotic" on the pack (or make your own! For a recipe, see *Love Your Gut*). I also recommend using yogurt with no added sugar, sweeteners, thickeners, or emulsifiers —just straight up full-fat (whole) milk and live cultures. Why full-fat? Studies have suggested that the fat can help the bacteria survive through our acidic stomachs. And remember, fat is not to be feared. It gives yogurt an amazing mouthfeel, prevents ice crystals from forming when freezing (such as in the Mango and Berry Froyo Bars on page 148) and can keep you satisfied for longer.

Salt and pepper

Because our taste buds adapt to our use of seasoning, the addition of salt in particular is very personal. I've only specified exact amounts of salt and pepper in the ingredients list where a precise amount is necessary. Otherwise, I've included salt and pepper in the ingredient list, along with a note in the method to "season to taste." For me, adding a little salt and pepper really does elevate a dish and adding a little salt to your cooking is fine for most (although if you have high blood pressure, it's worth reviewing your intake). When it comes to salt, I like to use sea salt, purely based on taste and texture. Despite the myths, it's not any "healthier."

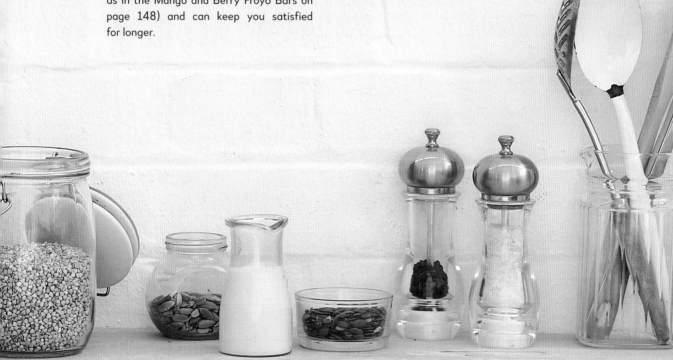

Breakfast

Muffin in a Mug

Plant Points
4.25

Serves **2**   Prep **3 minutes**   Cook **1.5 minutes per muffin**

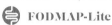 **FODMAP-Lite**

Looking after your gut health doesn't mean chocolatey goodness is off the breakfast menu. For those mornings when a bowl of cereal just won't cut it, this chocolate muffin is packed with hidden goodies for your gut microbes, including **9 grams of fiber per portion** and no added sugar. And it's ready in minutes . . . what's not to love?

2 large eggs

1 ripe banana

¼ cup (65 g) black beans, drained and rinsed

3 Medjool dates, pitted

½ cup (45 g) rolled oats

2 tablespoons cocoa powder

1 teaspoon baking powder

1 teaspoon vanilla extract

2 squares dark chocolate (about 0.35 ounce/10 g, optional)

¼ cup (60 g) probiotic yogurt, to serve

1. Crack the eggs into a high-powered blender and blend for 20 seconds. Add the banana, beans, dates, oats, cocoa powder, baking powder, and vanilla extract and blend for a further 20 seconds until smooth. Divide into two clean, microwave-safe cups (about 1 cup/240 ml capacity). Top with the chocolate (if using), then place one mug in the center of the microwave.

2. Cook on high for 1½ to 2 minutes, or until the muffin is set on top (it will keep cooking a little as it cools). Repeat with the second mug if cooking for two, or keep it in the fridge for tomorrow.

3. Allow to cool for a minute, then add a dollop of yogurt (if using) and enjoy.

Storage You can use your leftover black beans for the Loaded Vegan Nachos on page 233—or they can be kept in the fridge (in a sealed container, not the can) for up to 5 days.

Omelet Bowl

Plant Points
4.25

Serves **1**   Prep **2 minutes**   Cook **3 minutes**

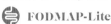 **FODMAP-Lite**

My "running late for a meeting but craving a savory breakfast" take on the humble Aussie zucchini slice, a favorite from my childhood. A hybrid between an omelet and a frittata with almost 7 grams of fiber, it's a deliciously healthy and easy way to start your day.

2 large eggs, beaten
½ zucchini, grated
1 slice seeded bread, torn into small pieces
⅓ cup (50 g) frozen peas
0.8 ounces (25 g) feta or cheese of choice, crumbled
1 tablespoon pine nuts (optional)
¼ teaspoon onion powder

1. Combine the eggs, zucchini, bread, peas, feta, pine nuts (if using), and onion powder in a microwave-safe dish.

2. Microwave on high for 2 minutes. Stir and heat for 1 more minute. If the eggs are still runny, continue to microwave in 20-second bursts until just set; it will keep cooking a little as it cools. Don't worry if it puffs up a lot in the microwave—it will sink back down.

3. Allow to cool for a minute before digging in.

Switch If you've already had zucchini and peas this week, swap them for 1 cup (about 130 g) frozen mixed vegetables of choice.

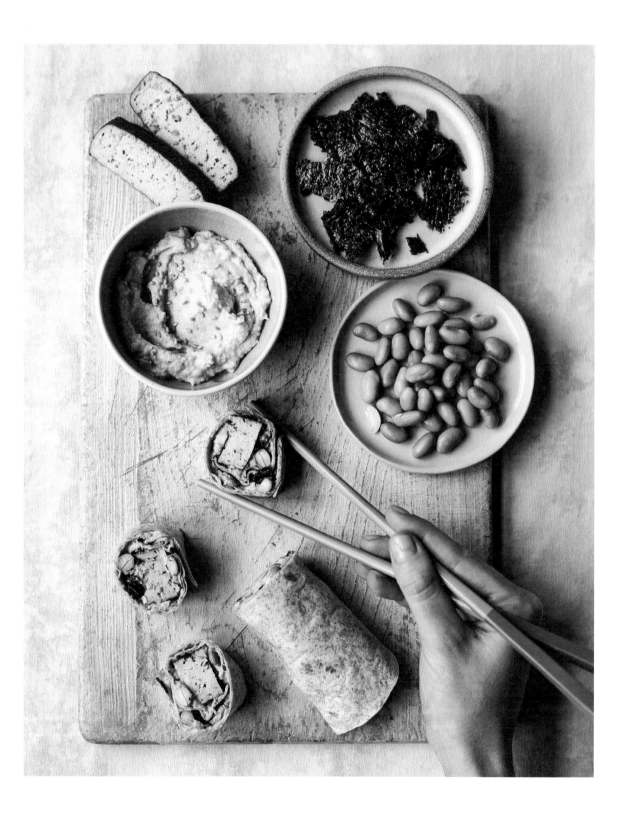

Fiber-Filled Breakfast Wrap

Plant Points
6.25

Makes **1 wrap**   Prep **5 minutes**

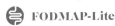 **FODMAP-Lite**

Inspired by Japanese norimaki sushi, where rice and fillings are placed in seaweed (nori) and rolled (maki), this recipe offers an impressive 12 grams of fiber per portion—that's around four times your traditional nori roll. Spread, sprinkle, wrap, and go!

3.5 ounces (100 g) smoked tofu
½ avocado
2 teaspoons probiotic yogurt or vegan aioli (see Garlicky Aquafaba Aioli, page 172)
1 teaspoon sesame oil
1 teaspoon sesame seeds
¼ teaspoon wasabi paste (optional)
1 whole grain wrap or wrap of choice
Sea salt
Fresh ground black pepper
⅓ cup (40 g) edamame beans, fresh, canned, or frozen
½ nori sheet, crumbled (optional)

1. Cut the tofu into two ¾-inch (2 cm) wide rectangles and set aside.

2. Mash together the avocado, yogurt, sesame oil, sesame seeds, and wasabi (if using) in a small bowl. Taste, season to preference, and then spread the mixture all over the wrap. Sprinkle the edamame and crumbled nori (if using) on top.

3. Lay the tofu along one edge of the wrap and then roll to encase it.

4. Cut into five pieces, about 1-inch (2.5 cm) wide, and enjoy.

Tip Can't find smoked tofu? Make your own by frying firm tofu in sesame oil for 2 to 3 minutes on each side. Prefer a warm breakfast? Heat the tofu strips and edamame beans in the microwave for 1 minute before layering them onto the wrap.

Switch Prefer a lighter breakfast? Switch out the whole grain wrap for a sheet of nori seaweed.

No-Bake Fruit and Nut Bites

Plant Points
12.5

Makes **12 balls or 4 breakfast bars**   Prep **15 minutes**

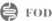 **FODMAP-Lite**   **Freezer**

On-the-go breakfast bites with a hit of fruit, veggies, whole grains, nuts, and seeds. These are ideal to make ahead of time, freeze, and then grab as you're running out the door in the morning. Unlike dense and overly sweet energy balls, this lighter version—delivering over a third of your daily fiber needs—will keep you and your microbes satisfied for longer.

11 dried apricots
½ cup (45 g) rolled oats
⅓ cup (30 g) unsweetened
    shredded coconut
2 tablespoons almond butter or nut
    butter of choice
1 tablespoon mixed seeds
1 teaspoon ground cinnamon
½ teaspoon ground ginger (optional)
1 carrot, grated
½ small apple, grated

Toppings (optional)
⅓ cup (30 g) unsweetened
    shredded coconut
¼ cup (25 g) mixed nuts, crushed

1. Place the apricots, oats, coconut, almond butter, mixed seeds, cinnamon, and ginger in a food processor and process for 1 minute or until well combined. Add in the carrot and apple and pulse a few times to roughly combine.

2. Divide the mix into 12 portions to make bites and 4 portions to make breakfast bars. Use your hands to shape each one into a ball or bar, and then roll the them in shredded coconut, nuts, or both (if using).

Storage These can be kept in the fridge for up to 5 days or in the freezer for up to 3 months.

DIY Plant-Packed Granola

Plant Points
18.5

Makes **20 servings**   Prep **10 minutes**   Bake **35 minutes**

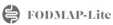 **FODMAP-Lite**

An essential for every pantry, this is best made at the start of the week so you can just pour it into a bowl and dive in on those busy weekdays.

²⁄₃ cup (100 g) quinoa
2½ cup (250 g) rolled oats
1 cup (100 g) cereal flakes of choice (corn, rice, rye)
1¾ cup (100 g) coconut flakes, toasted
3.5 ounces (100 g) dried apple, chopped
3.5 ounces (100 g) dried goji berries
3.5 ounces (100 g) dried mango, chopped
1 cup (100 g) mixed nuts, roughly chopped
¾ cup (100 g) mixed seeds
8 Medjool dates, made into a paste (see page 136) or ½ cup (120 ml) sweetener
⅓ cup (90 ml) extra virgin olive oil

Toppings
2 parsnips or carrots, washed and coarsely grated (about 10 ounces/300 g)
2 teaspoons ground cinnamon
1 teaspoon ground ginger
One 15-ounce (425 g) can of chickpeas or legumes of choice, drained and rinsed

To Serve
Berries
Milk of choice
Probiotic yogurt

1. Preheat the oven to 350°F (180°C) and line two large baking sheets with parchment paper.

2. To make the toppings, place the parsnips on a kitchen towel and pat dry, then place them on one of the baking sheets and toss with the cinnamon and ginger. Spread the parsnips on the baking sheet so they don't touch. Repeat the drying process with the chickpeas, then spread them across the second sheet.

3. Place both sheets in the oven for 20 minutes, then toss the parsnips and chickpeas, and bake for an additional 15 minutes or until completely dried out. Remove from the oven and allow to cool to room temperature (ideally overnight). Be sure to dry them out completely, otherwise they will turn the flakes soft.

4. For the quinoa, heat a large saucepan over medium-high heat. Once hot, add the quinoa in a single layer. Shake it over the heat until the quinoa starts to pop (a few minutes), but be careful not to let them burn. They won't pop dramatically like popcorn but will become tender and deliciously nutty. Allow to cool completely.

5. Mix the oats, cereal flakes, coconut flakes, apple, goji berries, mango, mixed nuts, and mixed seeds in a large bowl. Fold in the cooled parsnips, chickpeas, and quinoa.

6. Combine the date paste and olive oil in a bowl before adding the mixture. Using clean hands, toss to coat the granola, then spread it across the baking sheets.

7. Place in the oven for 10 minutes, toss, then bake for an additional 10 minutes or until crisp and golden. Allow to cool completely, then transfer to an airtight container.

8. Serve with berries, milk, and/or yogurt.

Storage Keep in an airtight container in a cool, dark place for up to 2 weeks.

Plant Points 7.5

Crispy Bacon-Shrooms with Creamy Butter Bean Hummus

Serves **2**   Prep **20 minutes**   Cook **20 minutes**

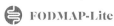 **FODMAP-Lite**

I created this recipe to show bacon-lovers that plants can be just as flavorful. The smoky, crunchy mushroom pieces, paired with the creamy butter bean hummus, really hit the spot— just ask my meat-loving husband. With 50 percent of your daily fiber needs per portion, you'll be well on your way to smashing your fiber goals.

Bacon-Shrooms
1 tablespoon red miso paste
1½ teaspoons soy sauce
1½ teaspoons Worcestershire sauce
1 Medjool date, made into a paste (see page 136), or 1 tablespoon sweetener
2 portobello mushrooms, roughly diced

Butter Bean Hummus
One 15-ounce (425 g) can butter beans, drained, and rinsed
¼ cup (60 ml) extra virgin olive oil, plus more to taste
3 tablespoons tahini
1 garlic clove
Juice of ½ lemon (about 1½ tablespoons), or to taste
1 tablespoon nutritional yeast (optional)
Sea salt
Fresh ground black pepper

To Serve
16 cherry tomatoes, ideally on the vine
¾ cup (50 g) roughly chopped kale
1 teaspoon extra virgin olive oil
4 slices seedy sourdough or bread of choice
Sea salt
Fresh ground black pepper

1. Preheat the oven to 425°F (220°C) and line two baking sheets with parchment paper.

2. To make the bacon-shrooms, mix the miso paste, soy sauce, Worcestershire sauce, and date paste in a medium bowl. Add the mushrooms and coat them well with the marinade. Spread the mushrooms out on one of the baking sheets and drizzle with any leftover marinade, then roast for 20 minutes, stirring after 10 minutes.

3. While the mushrooms are in the oven, place the butter beans, half the olive oil, tahini, and garlic with half the lemon juice in a food processor. Process to a smooth paste, then slowly add in the rest of the oil until you reach your preferred consistency. Stir in the nutritional yeast, then add more lemon juice and salt and pepper to taste. Set aside.

4. Place the tomatoes and kale on the other lined baking sheet, drizzle with olive oil, and season to taste. When the mushrooms are nearly cooked, place the kale and tomatoes in the oven and bake for 5 minutes, until the kale is just starting to crisp and the tomatoes are softening a little. The kale cooks very quickly, so keep an eye on it.

5. Toast the sourdough, spread with some of the butter bean hummus, and top with the bacon-shrooms, kale, and tomatoes.

Storage Store any leftover hummus in an airtight container in the fridge for up to 5 days. It's great as a dip or in sandwiches.

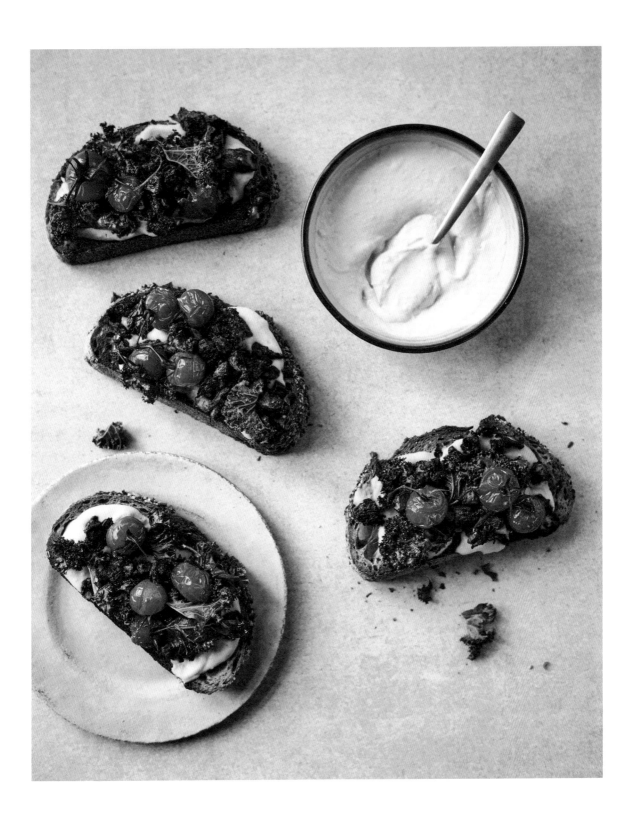

Mango and Berry Froyo Bars

Plant Points 5.25

Serves **6**   Prep **10 minutes, plus freezing**

 FODMAP-Lite   **Freezer**   **Zero Waste**

A gut-loving twist on your standard granola and yogurt breakfast, this recipe can be made as a bar or an ice pop. It's a perfect refreshing breakfast and makes a great summertime snack.

2 cups (300 g) frozen mixed berries or berries of choice
3⅓ cups (800 g) probiotic yogurt
2⅔ cups (400 g) frozen mango
3 large very ripe bananas, frozen
1 teaspoon ground turmeric
1½ cups (185 g) no-added-sugar granola (see DIY Plant-Packed Granola, page 145)

1. Line a 8 x 12 x 2-inch (20 x 30 x 5 cm) baking dish with parchment paper or prepare your ice pop molds.

2. Place the berries in the bottom of the dish (or molds) and mash them a little with a fork. Place the yogurt, mango, banana, and turmeric in a high-powered blender and blend for 30 seconds or until smooth.

3. Pour the mixture into the tray over the berries, and level it out with a spoon or spatula. Sprinkle the granola on top, gently pressing it down into the mix to make sure it sticks when it freezes.

4. Place in the freezer immediately to prevent the semi-frozen mix from melting (this will help prevent ice crystals from forming) and chill (ideally overnight) until fully set.

5. To serve, remove from the freezer 10 minutes beforehand, to allow the bars to soften a little. Use the paper to lift out the slab and cut into portions before digging in.

Storage Freeze the individual portions in an airtight container between layers of parchment paper for up to 2 weeks.

Tip Why full-fat yogurt? The fat not only protects the microbes as they travel through your acidic stomach, but it also makes for a creamier base.

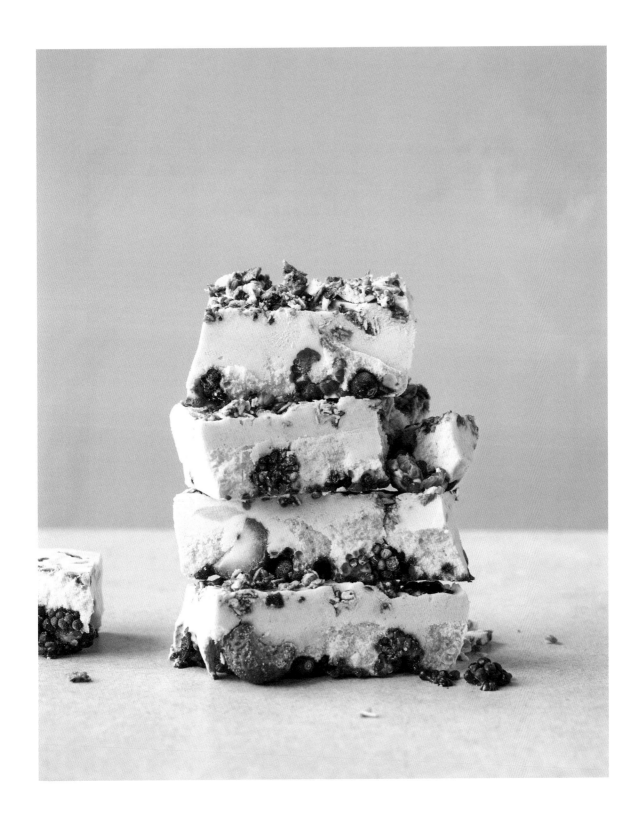

Plant-Powered Baked Oat Bars

Plant Points
11.5

Makes **8 to 10 slices**   Prep **15 minutes**   Cook **50 minutes**

 FODMAP-Lite   **Fridge Raid**   **Freezer**

My favorite on-the-go bar, loaded with prebiotics, plant points, and double the fiber of most breakfast slices. I make a batch at the start of the week and wrap up individual portions, so they're ready to grab as I'm heading out the door. Hearty, moist, and oh-so-satisfying alongside my morning cashew latte (see Frothy Cashew Latte, page 302).

One 15-ounce (425 g) can of cannellini beans, drained and rinsed

3 very ripe bananas

2 Medjool dates, made into a paste (see page 136) or 2 tablespoons sweetener

1¼ cup (300 ml) soy milk or milk of choice

2 cups (200 g) rolled oats

2 carrots (about 5 ounces/140 g), grated

1 cup (150 g) frozen raspberries or berry of choice

⅓ cup (50 g) raisins or dried fruit of choice

3 tablespoons dark chocolate chips

2 tablespoons flaxseed meal

1 tablespoon ground cinnamon

2 teaspoons vanilla extract

Olive oil, for greasing

1 tablespoon mixed seeds (optional)

1. Preheat the oven to 400°F (200°C).

2. Place the beans, bananas, date paste, and half the milk in a food processor and process until roughly blended (30 to 45 seconds). Transfer to a large bowl and stir in the oats, carrots, ⅔ cup raspberries, raisins, chocolate chips, flaxseed, cinnamon, and vanilla extract.

3. Lightly grease a rimmed baking sheet (9 x 13 x 1-inch/23 x 33 x 2.5 cm) and pour in the mix. Sprinkle over the reserved ⅓ cup (50 g) raspberries and mixed seeds (if using) and gently press them down into the mix.

4. Bake for 45 to 50 minutes, until the bars are golden brown and the berries have started to burst. Cover with foil toward the end if over-browning.

5. Allow to fully cool before serving or storing.

Switch Already had carrots this week? Replace them with 5 ounces (140 g) zucchini.

Storage These bars can be kept in the fridge for up to 4 days or in the freezer for up to 3 months. Cut into individual portions before freezing.

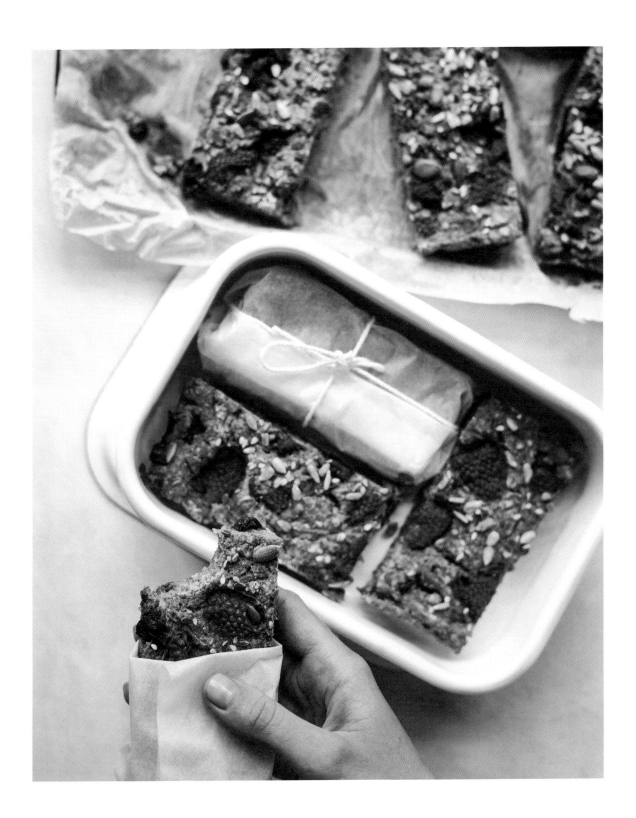

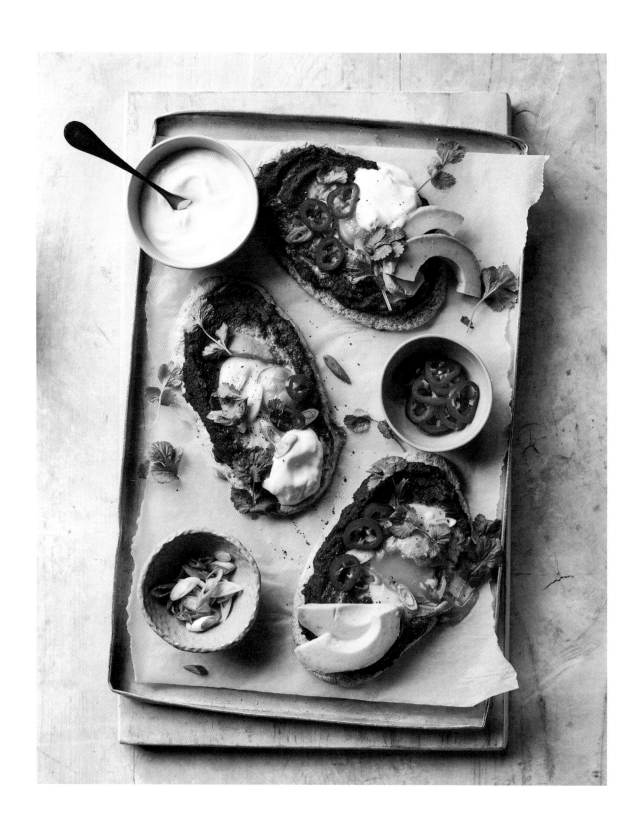

Breakfast Pita Pizza

Plant Points
5.5

Serves **4**   Prep **10 minutes**   Cook **8 minutes**

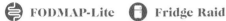 **FODMAP-Lite**   **Fridge Raid**

Who doesn't love the idea of pizza for breakfast? With a rich and tomatoey prebiotic base, this high-fiber pizza (boasting 12 g per pizza!) goes perfectly with a gooey egg and any leftover greens from the night before.

4 whole wheat pitas

Tomato Sauce
Half a 15-ounce (425 g) can kidney
    beans
10 sun-dried tomato halves, preserved
    in oil
2 ounces (60 g) pickled beets with
    3 tablespoons brine
1 scallion, roughly chopped
Sea salt
Fresh ground black pepper

Toppings
4 large eggs
3 tablespoons probiotic yogurt
1 avocado, sliced
1 scallion, finely chopped
⅓ cup (10 g) chopped fresh cilantro
1 red chile, sliced

Other Topping Suggestions
Capers
Flaked salmon
Leftover cooked veggies
Mackerel
Mixed greens
Olives
Parmesan shavings
Peppers
Pine nuts

1. Preheat the oven to 475°F (250°C). Line a baking sheet with parchment paper.

2. Lay the pitas on the baking sheet.

3. Place the kidney beans, sun-dried tomatoes, beets, and scallion in a food processor and blend to form a smooth paste. Use a splash of water to thin it out if needed.

4. Spread a quarter of the tomato sauce over each of the pitas, with a thicker layer around the edge to prevent the egg from sliding off. Crack an egg into the center of each pita.

5. Place the baking sheet in the oven for 8 to 10 minutes, until the eggs are cooked to your liking. Remove from the oven and add toppings. Season to taste.

Storage Any leftover tomato sauce can be used as a dip, a spread for sandwiches, a sauce for pasta, and more. Store in an airtight container in the fridge for up to 5 days.

Switch I tend to add leftover cooked veggies, but if you've only got raw, add a drizzle of olive oil to a large frying pan over medium-high heat and cook for 5 minutes until the veggies start to soften. This helps to remove some of the moisture, saving you from a wet pizza. Add the veggies and any other toppings that you prefer warm to your pita before placing it in the oven.

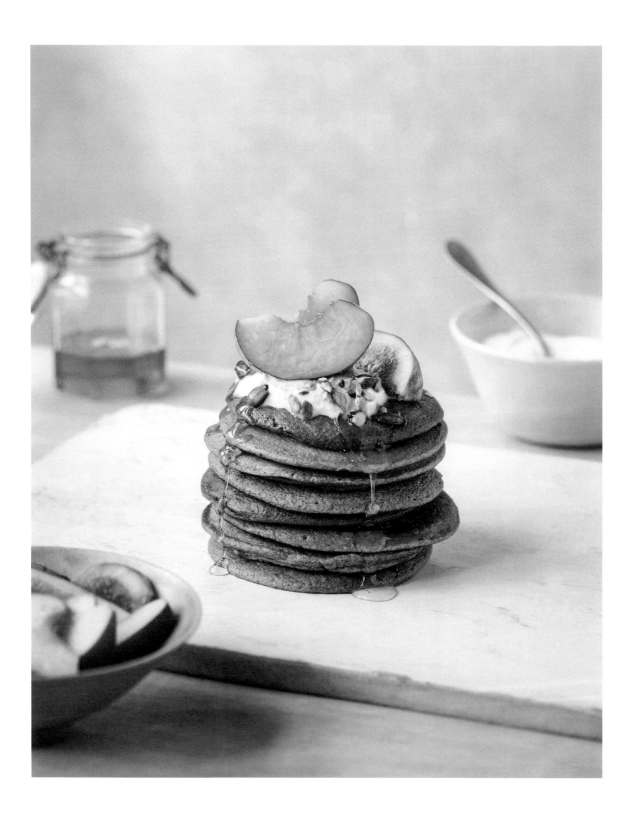

Eat-the-Rainbow Pancakes

Plant Points
8.25

Makes **8 small pancakes of one color**   Prep **5 minutes**   Cook **15 minutes**

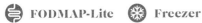

🌀 **FODMAP-Lite**   ❄️ **Freezer**

Nature features so many amazing colors, and this family-favorite breakfast celebrates just that. Alongside the array of gut-loving phytochemicals with their brilliant tones, these rainbow pancakes have just four simple base ingredients and not a food dye in sight. Ease, taste, and gut-love all in one!

Batter
2 ripe bananas
2 large eggs
½ cup (45 g) rolled oats
Extra virgin olive oil, for frying

Colorings (choose 1 per batch)
a. *Pretty Pink (betalain)*
    ½ small beet (1 ounce/28 g)
b. *Mellow Yellow (curcumin)*
    1 teaspoon turmeric
c. *Proud Purple (anthocyanin)*
    ½ cup (40 g) shredded red cabbage
d. *Go Green (chlorophyll)*
    1 cup (30 g) baby spinach leaves

Toppings (optional)
Berries, whole or pureed
Fresh figs
Grilled banana
Probiotic yogurt, sweetened with honey
Toasted mixed seeds

1. Place the bananas, oats, and eggs along with one of the plant colorings, in a high-powered blender. Blend for 1 to 2 minutes, until smooth and a little foamy on top.

2. If you are making additional batches using different colorings (as I've done in the image on the previous page), pour the first batch into a jug and set aside. Rinse the blender and repeat the step above.

3. Heat the olive oil in a large frying pan (or two) over low heat, before spooning in about 3 tablespoons of the batter per pancake.

4. Cook for 2 to 3 minutes, until you see the top of the pancake start to bubble and dry around the edges. Flip and cook the other side for another few minutes. Don't be tempted to increase the heat level; if you do, you'll lose the vibrant colors.

5. Repeat until you've used up all the batter. Enjoy with toppings of your choice.

Storage   These are best eaten right away, but they can be kept in the fridge for 3 days or frozen for up to 1 month layered between pieces of parchment paper in an airtight container.

Sweet
Treats

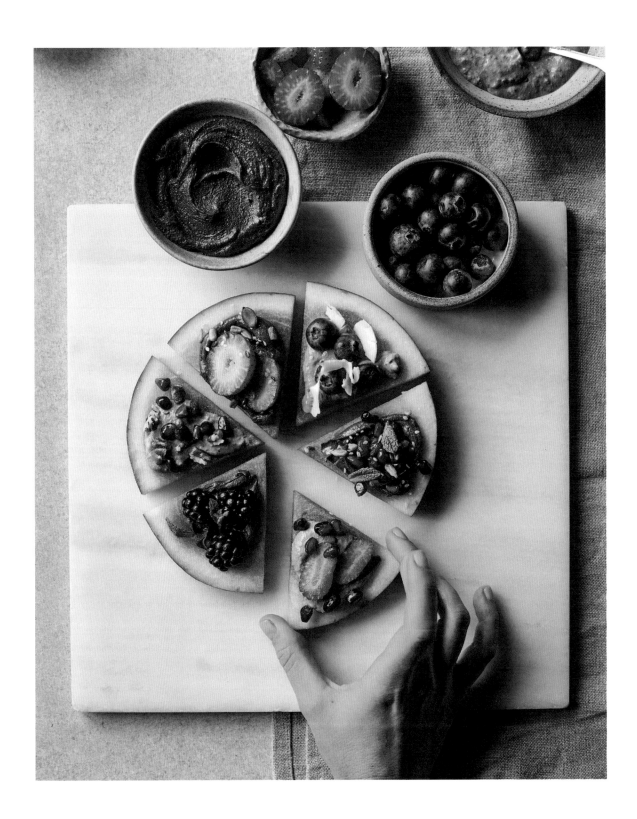

Loaded Melon Wedges

Plant Points
9.5

Serves **4**   Prep **10 minutes**   Cook **10 minutes**

 FODMAP-Lite   **Fridge Raid**

Turn snack time into a fun family activity that brings everyone together to create their own watermelon masterpiece. Get creative with the toppings to celebrate the bursting colors of plants and the indulgent flavors of cocoa and hazelnuts.

2 large watermelon slices or melon
   of choice (about 1 inch/2.5 cm thick)

Berry Whip Spread
⅔ cup (100 g) blackberries (or about
   16 pitted cherries)
Scant ½ cup (100 g) ricotta
Honey, to taste (optional)

Chocolate-Hazelnut Spread
1½ cups (200 g) hazelnuts
3.5 ounces (100 g) dark chocolate
   (at least 70 percent)
1 teaspoon vanilla extract

Toppings (optional)
Blueberries
Coconut flakes
Fresh herb leaves (like mint)
Mixed seeds
Pecans
Pomegranate seeds
Strawberries

1. Cut each slice of watermelon into 6 to 8 triangles, depending on the size of your watermelon.

2. To make the berry whip spread, place the berries, ricotta, and honey (if using) in a blender and blend until smooth. Set aside.

3. To make the chocolate-hazelnut spread, preheat the oven to 350°F (180°C). Spread the hazelnuts out on a baking sheet and roast for 5 minutes until lightly golden. While the nuts are in the oven, break the chocolate into pieces and place in a heatproof bowl. Melt by either placing over a saucepan of simmering water or heating in a microwave in 30-second bursts.

4. Place the hazelnuts in a high-powered food processor. Blend for 10 to 15 minutes until a smooth nut butter has formed. Scrape in the melted chocolate and add the vanilla extract. Blend for another few seconds until well combined and glossy.

5. Top the melon wedges with either spread, along with your choice of toppings.

Tip Keep your watermelon in the fridge before serving for an extra-refreshing slice.

Storage The berry whip spread keeps in the fridge for up to 24 hours and the chocolate-hazelnut spread for up to 2 weeks in an airtight jar.

Fruit and Nut Wheels

Plant Points
10

Makes **18 wheels**   Prep **15 minutes**   Chill **4 hours**

 Freezer

This glossy fruit log is packed full of plant diversity—with fruits, nuts, and seeds all rolled up into one delicious package. It's one of my favorite recipes to show that plant-based doesn't mean boring. It's also a great way to diversify high-fiber snacks for kids, and chances are you already have the ingredients in your pantry.

20 apricots

13 dried figs

⅓ cup (40 g) pistachios, roughly chopped

¼ cup (25 g) walnuts, roughly chopped

2 tablespoons mixed seeds

¼ cup (25 g) almond meal

¼ cup (15 g) coconut flakes

1 tablespoon dried cranberries

2 tablespoons unsweetened shredded coconut (optional)

1. Place the apricots and figs in a food processor and blend into a thick paste. It will take 1 to 2 minutes and you may need to scrape the sides down.

2. Place the pistachios, walnuts, and mixed seeds in a dry frying pan over medium heat. Toast for 2 to 3 minutes, stirring regularly to prevent burning.

3. Transfer the fruit paste to a large bowl along with the almond meal, coconut flakes, cranberries and, once cooled, the pistachios, walnuts, and seeds. Mix with your hands, pressing and turning the mixture repeatedly to help coax it together.

4. On a clean work surface, lay out a long piece of plastic wrap. Shape the mixture into a log about 2 inches (5 cm) in diameter. Sprinkle the shredded coconut (if using) onto the plastic wrap and roll the log until coated.

5. Wrap the log tightly in the plastic wrap, twisting the ends to make it airtight, and pop it in the freezer to harden for at least 4 hours. To serve, unwrap it (while still frozen) and use a sharp knife to cut it into 18 mini-wheels.

6. I love eating the wheels straight from the freezer, but store in the fridge if you prefer a softer texture. Enjoy!

Storage   Store in the fridge in an airtight container for up to 2 weeks or in the freezer for up to 2 months.

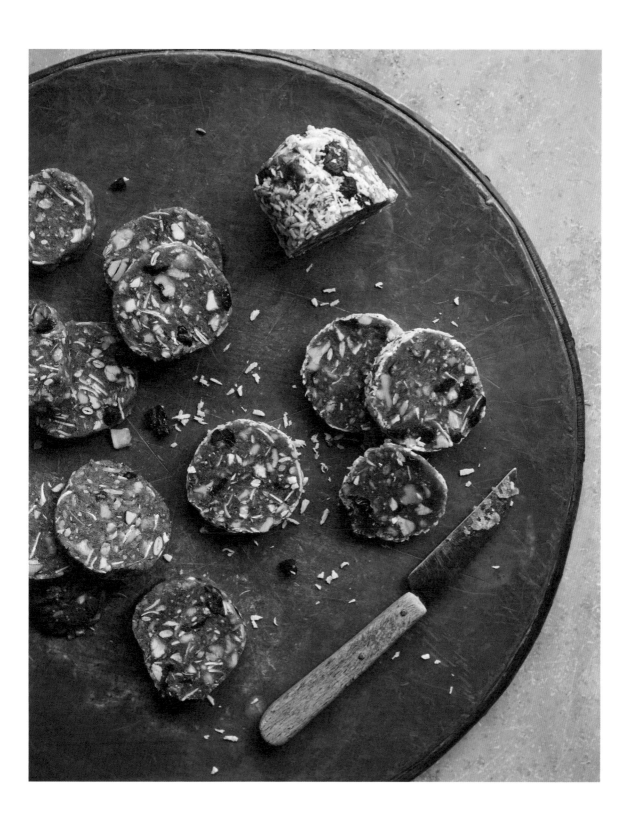

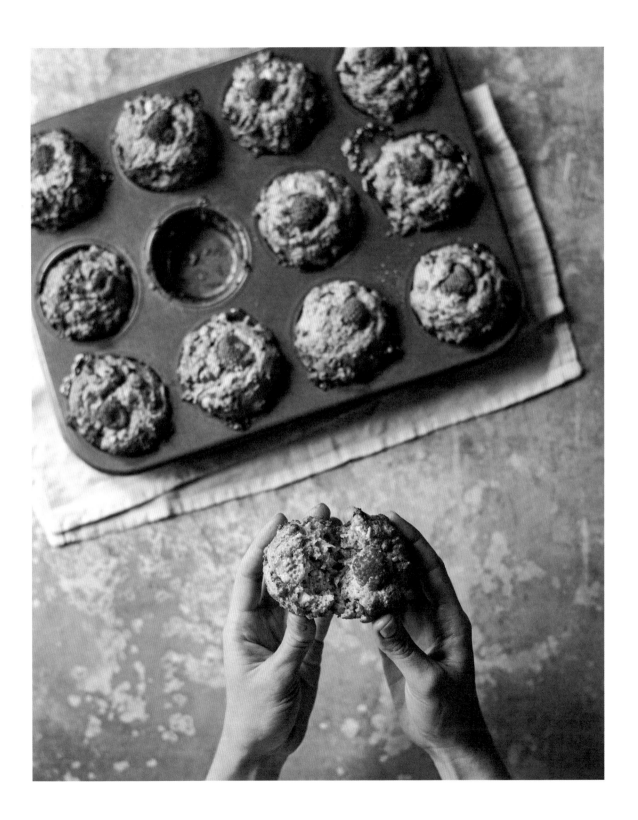

Ultimate Raspberry and White Chocolate Muffins

Plant Points
5.5

Makes **12 muffins**   Prep **15 minutes**   Cook **25 minutes**

 FODMAP-Lite   **Freezer**

Inspired by the muffins I used to get from my local bakery, these muffins combine my two favorite things: white chocolate and plants! The raspberries are a top source of gut-loving polyphenols, too. What's more satisfying than a sweet, moist muffin and knowing that you're 5.5 plant points closer to your 30 for the week?

3 large eggs, beaten

⅔ cup (160 g) probiotic yogurt

1 very ripe banana

¼ cup (60 ml) extra virgin olive oil, plus more for greasing

3 Medjool dates, pitted and roughly chopped or 3 tablespoons sweetener of choice

2 teaspoons vanilla extract

2¼ cup (270 g) spelt flour or whole wheat flour

2 teaspoons baking powder

⅔ cup (100 g) white chocolate chips

1 tablespoon poppy seeds

2 carrots (about 5 ounces/140 g), shredded

⅔ cup (100 g) frozen raspberries

To Decorate

12 raspberries, frozen or fresh

1. Preheat the oven to 375°F (190°C). Grease a 12-cup muffin pan and add a disc of parchment paper to the bottom of each to prevent sticking.

2. Place the eggs in a food processor and blend for 30 seconds, until a little foamy. Add in the yogurt, banana, olive oil, dates, and vanilla extract and blend for 30 seconds or until smooth.

3. In a large bowl, mix together the flour and baking powder, then stir in the chocolate chips and poppy seeds. Pour in the wet mixture from the food processor, followed by the carrots and raspberries. Combine to form a thick batter.

4. Fill each muffin cup evenly with batter. Push one raspberry into the top of each muffin, then place the pan in the oven.

5. Bake the muffins for 25 to 30 minutes, until a skewer comes out clean (minus any melted white chocolate), then place the muffins on a wire rack to cool before digging in!

Storage These can be kept in an airtight container for 3 days or frozen for up to 3 months.

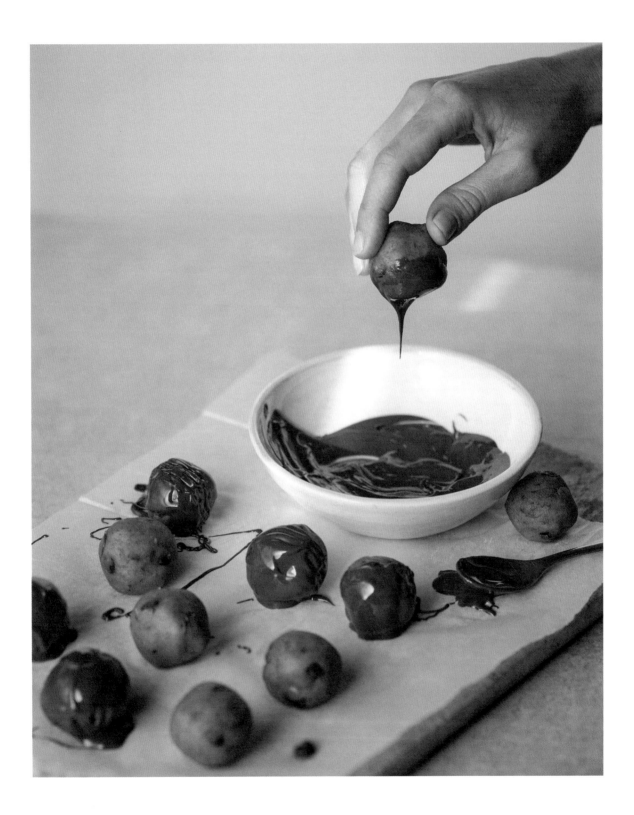

Prebiotic Cookie Dough Drops

Plant Points
4.25

Makes **12 drops**   Prep **10 minutes**

❄️ **Freezer**

Raw cookie dough reminds me of baking with my granny, so I wanted to recreate it with a version that I could also share with my gut microbes. This is a perfect afternoon pick-me-up, boasting **4.25** plant points in every ball. It's also an ideal treat for a movie night. Try it in your favorite ice cream.

Half of a 15-ounce (425 g) can chickpeas, drained and rinsed twice

5 Medjool dates, pitted and roughly chopped

⅓ cup (80 g) cashew butter (see below) or nut or seed butter of choice

3 tablespoons almond meal

1 teaspoon vanilla extract

3 tablespoons dark chocolate chips, roughly chopped

3 ounces (85 g) chocolate of choice for coating (optional)

1. Line a baking sheet with parchment paper.

2. Place the chickpeas, dates, nut butter, almond meal, and vanilla extract in a food processor and blend for 1 to 2 minutes to form a thick paste. If the mixture is a little dry, add some water to help it blend (a bit at a time, up to 1 tablespoon). Stir in the chocolate chips.

3. Divide the dough into 12 even pieces and roll into balls. Place the balls onto the baking sheet and chill in the fridge while you melt the chocolate (if using).

4. Break the chocolate into pieces and place in a heatproof mixing bowl. Melt by either placing over a saucepan of simmering water or heating in the microwave in 30-second bursts.

5. Decorate the drops with as much of the chocolate as you like— dunk fully, drizzle, or pour a spoonful over. The cookie dough is also delicious on its own!

Homemade Nut Butter

Makes about ⅔ cup (160 g)

1¼ cups (165 g) cashews

Sea salt

1½ teaspoons extra virgin olive oil

Can't get your hands on cashew butter? Make your own!

1. Preheat the oven to 350°F (180°C).

2. Place the cashews on a baking sheet and bake for 5 minutes until golden and toasted. Remove from the oven and place in a food processor with the olive oil and sea salt. Blend for a few minutes until a nut butter forms, scraping down the sides occasionally. As the cashews blend, they transform into a powder, then a clumpy mix, and finally a smooth butter.

Tip You can also try putting some of the cookie dough into the ice cream recipe on page 279. Just break it into pieces and stir through before freezing.

Storage The balls will keep for up to 1 week in the fridge or up to 1 month in the freezer.

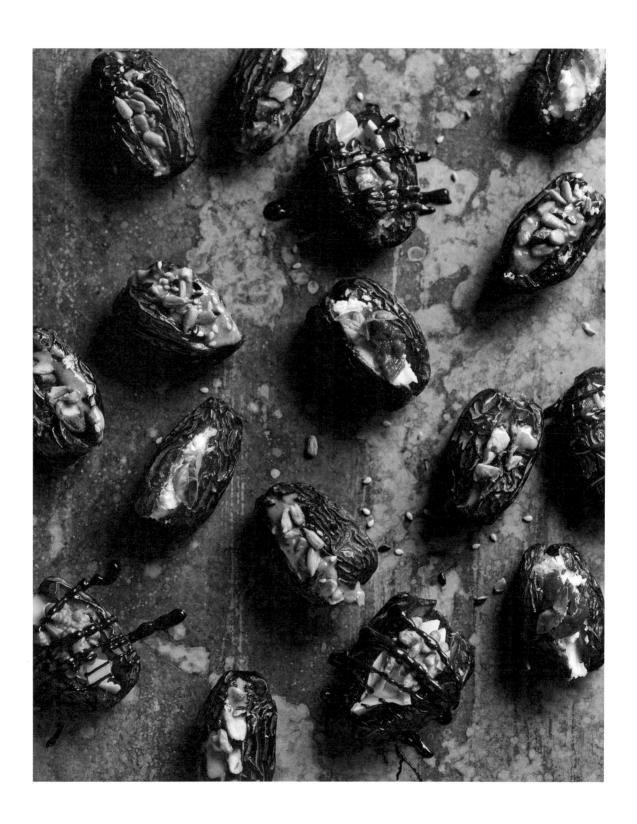

Stuffed Dates, Four Ways

Plant Points
2.25

Serves **1**   Prep **2 minutes**

 Freezer

I like to think of dates as nature's high-fiber sweeties, since their chewy sweetness feels so indulgent. They're my go-to for a quick treat, filled with my favorite flavor combos. Feel free to experiment with your own filling ideas, too. They're also great for freezing—if you have any left, that is!

1 pitted Medjool date

Sweet and Salty
0.35 ounce (10 g) goat cheese
1 basil leaf
1 sun-dried tomato half, preserved in oil

Seed 'n' Nut
1 heaping teaspoon nut butter of choice
Pinch of mixed seeds, toasted

Creamy Tahini
1 heaping teaspoon tahini
5 pistachios

Chocolate-Walnut
1 tablespoon coconut flakes
1 walnut
Drizzle of melted dark chocolate

1. Slice the date lengthwise, removing the pit to make a pocket.

2. Stuff your filling of choice into the pocket—it really is that simple!

Tip Pop your stuffed dates in the freezer for ready-to-go sweet treats all week—the freeze makes them even softer and creamier.

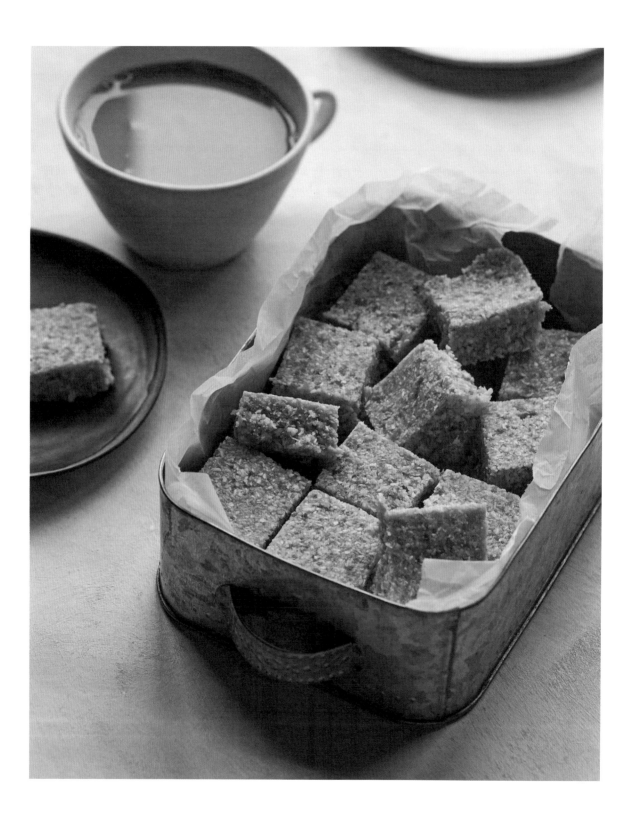

Four-Ingredient Citrus Bars

Plant Points
3

Makes **25 squares**   Prep **10 minutes**   Chill **30 minutes to 4 hours**

 Freezer

For those days when a piece of fruit won't cut it, but you're short on time for baking. Move over store-bought granola bars—this refreshing treat is the ultimate high-fiber accompaniment to a comforting cup of tea.

Scant 1½ cups (200 g) cashews
2½ cups (200 g) unsweetened
   shredded coconut
21 dried apricots (about 5 ounces/
   150 g)
Juice of 1 large orange (about ⅓ cup/
   80 ml), plus zest to taste

1. Line the base and sides of an 8-inch (20 cm) square baking pan with parchment paper.

2. Place the cashews in a food processor and blend for 30 seconds until ground. Add the coconut and apricots and pulse until the apricots are finely chopped. Add the orange juice and blend again until the mixture forms a ball, about 1 minute. Taste and add zest to preference.

3. Firmly press the mixture into the pan with the back of a spoon. Chill in the fridge for 4 hours (or in the freezer for 30 minutes) or until firm enough to cut. Slice into 25 squares.

Storage These will keep in the fridge for up to 5 days. Or you can freeze the sliced squares between pieces of parchment paper in an airtight container for up to 3 months.

Switch For an extra plant point, add a shredded carrot (about ¾ cup/75 g) and reduce the orange juice to ¼ cup (60 ml).

Light
Bites

Garlicky Aquafaba Aioli

Makes **1 cup (240 ml), eight 2-tablespoon portions**   Prep **15 minutes**

 FODMAP-Lite   **Zero Waste**

Like my grandad always used to say, "Waste not, want not." After you've tried this thick and creamy aioli, you'll never look at the too-often-discarded liquid from canned chickpeas the same way again. (Oh, and did you know the liquid contains prebiotics?) Not only is this aioli easy to make, it's also incredibly versatile and goes perfectly with my Smoky Beet Burgers (page 215), Snack-o-Clock Veggie Fritters (page 181), Popcorn Chick-less Nuggets (page 185), and just about everything else!

⅓ cup (80 ml) aquafaba from a 15-ounce (425 g) can of chickpeas, chilled
1½ to 2 teaspoons lemon juice, to taste
1 small garlic clove, grated or minced
Pinch of mustard powder
1 cup (240 ml) sunflower oil or any neutral vegetable oil such as canola or avocado
Sea salt
Fresh ground black pepper

1. Place the aquafaba, lemon juice, garlic, and mustard powder in a blender and blend for 1 minute.

2. Very slowly pour the oil into the blender while blending at high speed for 7 to 12 minutes, until the mixture becomes thick and creamy. If you pour in the oil too quickly, the mixture won't thicken.

3. Adjust the lemon juice and add salt and pepper to taste.

Storage Keep in the fridge in an airtight container for up to 2 weeks.

Creamy Pistachio Dip

Plant Points
3.75

Makes **1 cup (240 g), eight 2-tablespoon portions**   Prep **5 minutes**

 Freezer

Don't let the name limit this dip's true potential—it's also delicious stirred through pasta like a creamy pesto, and it pairs perfectly with my Foolproof Fermented Wheaten Bread (page 178) as a spread. You'll be scraping out every last bit.

4 cups (120 g) baby spinach
1 small avocado, halved
¼ cup (60 ml) extra virgin olive oil
½ cup (60 g) shelled pistachios
Juice of ½ to 1 lemon (1½ to
    3 tablespoons), to taste
1 cup (15 g) fresh basil
1 garlic clove
Sea salt
Fresh ground black pepper

Place all the ingredients in a food processor and blend for about 1 minute if you like a little texture or 3 minutes if you prefer a smooth dip. Adjust lemon juice and salt and pepper to taste.

Storage This will keep in an airtight container in the fridge for up to 1 week.

Tip To prevent the avocado from turning brown, cover the dip in a thin layer of extra virgin olive oil or press a piece of plastic wrap directly onto the dip and store it in the fridge. Why does the browning happen? It's all thanks to a chemical reaction known as oxidation, in which the air "reacts" with those beneficial polyphenols, producing melanin —the compound that pigments our skin.

Smoky Eggplant Dip

Plant Points
6.25

Makes **1 scant cup (225 g), seven 2-tablespoon portions**   Prep **10 minutes**   Cook **25 minutes**

 FODMAP-Lite   **Freezer**

Creamy, smoky eggplant is one of my favorite flavors, so I created this dip recipe, inspired by baba ghanoush. You can eat this with crunchy veggies, spread it on a seedy cracker (see Seedy Cracker Duo, page 177) or bread (see Foolproof Fermented Wheaten Bread, page 178), or serve it as a side alongside some roasted veggies and couscous. Did you know eggplant is a fruit? In fact, it's technically a large berry!

2 eggplants (about 21 ounces/600 g), halved lengthwise
1 garlic clove
Juice of 1 lemon (about 3 tablespoons), plus zest to taste
2 tablespoons tahini
1 tablespoon extra virgin olive oil
½ teaspoon ground cumin
½ teaspoon smoked paprika
Sea salt
Fresh ground black pepper
2 tablespoons capers, finely chopped (optional)

Toppings (optional)
1 tablespoon parsley, finely chopped
2 tablespoons pomegranate seeds
½ teaspoon sesame seeds

1. Preheat the grill and line a roasting pan with foil. Grease the foil with olive oil.

2. Place the eggplants, skin up, in the pan, and grill for 25 minutes or until the skin is fully charred. Add the garlic to roast for the final 5 minutes. Remove from the grill and leave until cool enough to handle.

3. Scoop out the eggplant flesh and place in a high-powered blender along with the roasted garlic. Add the lemon juice, tahini, olive oil, cumin, paprika, salt, and pepper, then blend until smooth.

4. Stir in the capers. Taste and adjust seasoning as needed.

5. Spoon into a bowl, and top with parsley, pomegranate seeds, and sesame seeds (if using).

Storage   This will keep in the fridge in an airtight container for 4 to 5 days.

No-Added-Sugar Ketchup

Plant Points
6.5

Makes **1 scant cup (225 g), fifteen 2-tablespoon portions**   Prep **15 minutes**   Cook **35 minutes**

 FODMAP-Lite   **Freezer**

This homemade ketchup packs that same flavor punch as the bottled stuff that many of us grew up on—but this one is full of diverse plant goodness without the added sugar. Perfect for dipping Popcorn Chick-less Nuggets (page 185) into.

1 teaspoon extra virgin olive oil
1 small red onion, chopped
½ cup (70 g) peeled, chopped butternut squash
1 small red apple, chopped
1 carrot, chopped
½ teaspoon sea salt
One 14.5-ounce (411 g) can diced tomatoes
1 teaspoon paprika
2 Medjool dates, pitted and roughly chopped
3 tablespoons tomato paste
3 tablespoons pickled beet juice, from a jar

1. Heat the olive oil in a saucepan over medium-low heat. Add the apple, onion, squash, carrot, and salt. Cover and cook until softened, about 15 minutes. If the mixture gets too dry, add 1 to 2 tablespoons of cold water.

2. Add the tomatoes, tomato paste, dates, and paprika. Turn the heat down to low, cover, and simmer until the vegetables have softened, 20 minutes.

3. Allow to cool, then transfer the mixture to a food processor along with the beet juice. Blend for 1 minute or until smooth, then adjust seasoning to taste.

Storage This will keep in the fridge for 1 week or frozen for up to 1 month.

Tip For some added microbes, add 1 tablespoon of sauerkraut juice before blending. Transfer to an airtight container and leave out of direct sunlight for 4 hours (to allow the microbes to begin their fermenting feast). Taste and adjust seasoning as needed before storing in the fridge.

Switch Prefer a smoky tomato sauce? Switch out the paprika for smoked paprika.

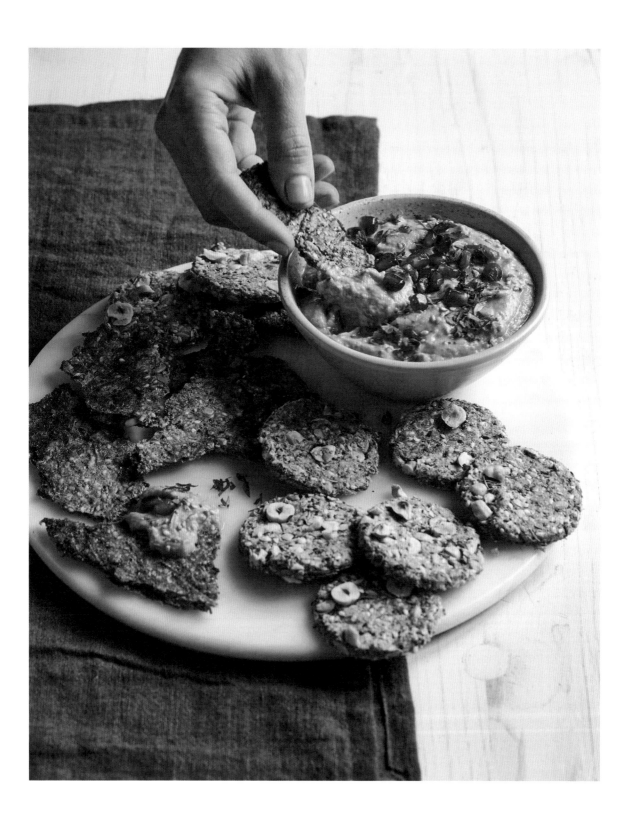

Plant Points
6.5

Seedy Cracker Duo

Serves **6 (about 3 crackers per portion)**   Prep **10 minutes**   Cook **25 minutes**

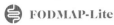 **FODMAP-Lite**

A pantry staple in my household. These crunchy crackers are the perfect delivery vehicle for a host of toppings when you need a quick bite between meals. They also serve up an impressive 4 grams of fiber per portion, which is more than four times as much as store-bought crackers.

Base
2 tablespoons flaxseed meal
⅓ cup plus 1 tablespoon (95 ml)
    boiling water
Scant 1 cup (120 g) mixed seeds
¾ cup (80 g) rye flour or flour of choice
2 tablespoons extra virgin olive oil

Flavors (choose one)
Roasted hazelnut
½ cup (65 g) hazelnuts, chopped
1 teaspoon dried thyme

Cheesy beet
¼ small beet (about 0.75 ounce/20 g),
    finely grated and patted dry
2 tablespoons nutritional yeast

1. Mix the flaxseed meal and water in a small bowl and set aside for 5 minutes to thicken.

2. Preheat the oven to 350°F (180°C) and line a baking sheet with parchment paper.

3. Choose your flavor. Mix the mixed seeds, flour, and olive oil in a medium bowl along with the hydrated flaxseed and the ingredients for your chosen flavor (if using the hazelnuts, mix in only half of them, leaving the remainder to press on top) and a big pinch of sea salt, to form a rough dough. Leave for a few minutes to thicken.

4. Transfer the dough to a sheet of parchment paper and place a second sheet over the top of the dough. Roll out the dough between the sheets of paper, as thin as you can get it. I roll mine paper-thin, for an extra-crispy cracker.

5. Sprinkle over a little extra sea salt to taste (if using the hazelnuts, scatter the remaining nuts on top and gently press them into the dough).

6. Use a 2.5-inch (6 cm) cookie cutter to cut out about 18 rounds and place them on the baking sheet, or go for the rustic look and bake the crackers in a whole sheet. Place in the oven and bake for 20 to 30 minutes, until crispy and golden.

7. Place on a wire rack to cool before lifting them from the paper.

Storage These will keep in an airtight container at room temperature for up to 2 weeks if fully dried out.

Foolproof Fermented Wheaten Bread

Plant Points
4.25

Makes **1 medium loaf (12 slices)** Prep **10 minutes (plus 3 hours for fermenting)** Cook **40 minutes**

❄ **Freezer**

After I fell in love with wheaten bread in Ireland, my father-in-law entrusted me with his foolproof recipe. With a few gut-loving tweaks here and there, I present to you this game-changing recipe. Crunchy crust with a deliciously moist and dense crumb—you'll never need to buy bread again.

2 cups (300 g) whole wheat flour, plus
    extra for dusting
Generous ¾ cup (200 g)
    probiotic yogurt
1 large carrot, shredded
1 tablespoon pumpkin seeds
1 tablespoon sesame seeds
1 teaspoon baking soda
3 thyme sprigs, leaves picked, or
    1 teaspoon dried thyme
½ teaspoon sea salt

Preheat the oven to 400°F (200°C).

Fermenting option:

Mix 1 cup (150 g) flour with the yogurt and ⅓ cup plus 1 tablespoon (100 ml) of water. Cover the bowl with a clean kitchen towel and leave to ferment for about 3 hours (out of direct sunlight). When ready to bake, mix in the carrot, pumpkin seeds, sesame seeds, baking soda, thyme, and salt, using a butter knife to combine. Be careful not to overwork the dough as this will make it tough.

Non-fermenting option:

Combine the flour, carrot, pumpkin seeds, sesame seeds, baking soda, thyme, and salt in a large bowl. Mix well. Add in the yogurt along with ⅓ cup plus 1 tablespoon (100 ml) of water and stir with a butter knife to make a soft sticky dough. Be careful not to overwork the dough.

To bake:

1. Gently turn the dough onto a lightly floured baking sheet and bring it together into a loaf shape. Score a cross on top with a sharp knife.

2. Bake for 40 to 50 minutes, until golden, and check that the base is dry and the loaf sounds hollow when tapped. Place on a wire rack and let it cool completely.

Storage Well wrapped, this bread will keep for 2 days at room temperature, 5 days in the fridge, or up to 3 months in the freezer. I freeze mine in individual portions so I always have a serving on hand (just defrost in the microwave for a minute).

Switch If you've already had carrots this week, the recipe also works with ⅔ cup (100 g) grated zucchini—just reduce the water to ⅓ cup (80 ml).

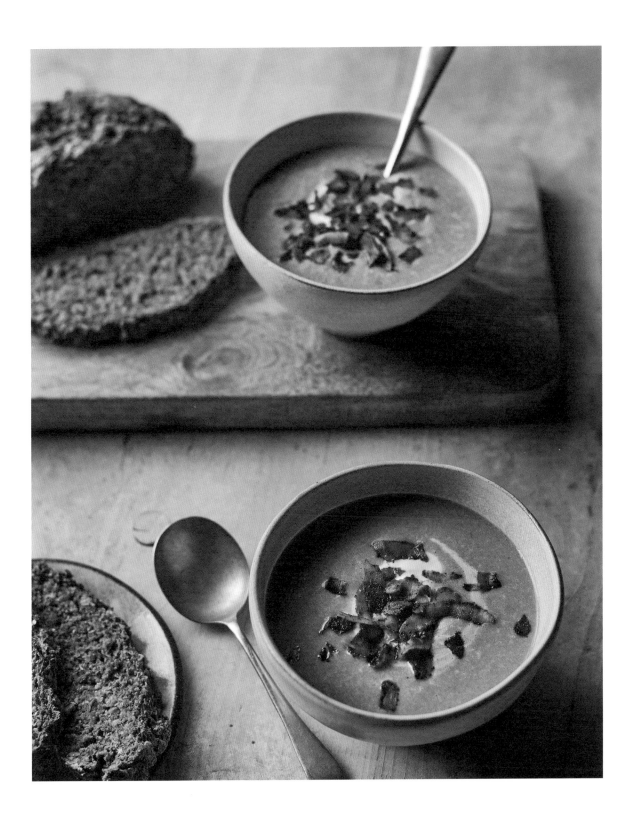

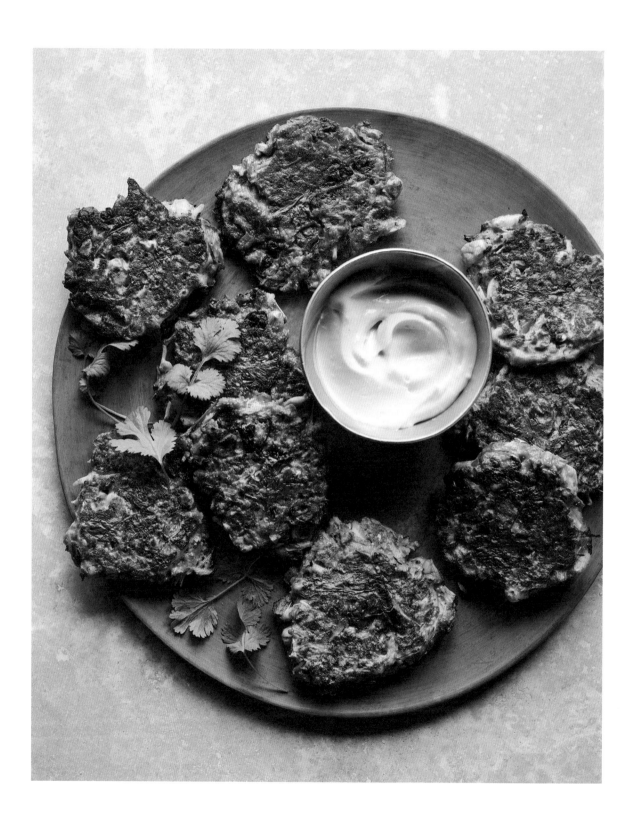

Snack-o-Clock Veggie Fritters

Plant Points
5.5

Makes **10 fritters**   Prep **10 minutes**   Cook **20 minutes**

🌀 **FODMAP-Lite**   🧊 **Fridge Raid**

Perfect for packing in your plant points and using up any leftover veggies in your fridge. I love pairing these with my Garlicky Aquafaba Aioli (page 172) or adding a side salad and some sweet potato wedges for a flavorful feast!

3 large eggs
4 cups (300 g) mixed sliced stir-fry vegetables (e.g., cabbage, carrots, onion)
⅔ cup (80 g) fava beans, fresh or canned
⅓ cup (50 g) whole wheat flour or flour of choice
2 tablespoons red miso
Fresh ground black pepper
2 tablespoons extra virgin olive oil
⅓ cup (10 g) fresh cilantro

1. Crack the eggs into a food processor and process for 12 seconds or so, until nice and fluffy. Add in the veggies and beans and blend for a few seconds to roughly break up the beans and any larger vegetable pieces.

2. Transfer to a large bowl. Add the flour, miso, and pepper to taste. Mix to form a thick batter.

3. Heat the oil in a large frying pan over medium heat. Once the pan is hot, add ¼ cup (60 g) of the batter into the pan for each fritter. Press a few cilantro leaves on to the surface of the batter.

4. Cover and fry until golden brown, 5 to 6 minutes, then flip and cook for 1 to 2 minutes more on the other side. Repeat until you've used all the batter. The fritters are delicate at first, so try not to peek at the bottoms for the first few minutes, until they start to crisp up.

5. Serve and enjoy warm—or put them in your lunch box for tomorrow!

Tip You can experiment with other types of miso (such as white miso) and you'll end up with a different-tasting fritter. White miso is sweeter, yellow miso is earthy, and red miso is packed with umami—yum!

Storage Leftover fritters can be kept in the fridge for 3 days.

Switch Want an extra plant point? Add in ⅔ cup (100 g) cooked or raw corn kernels and reduce the stir-fry veggies to 3 cups (200 g).

All-the-Greens Phyllo Pie

Plant Points
5.5

Serves **4** Prep **20 minutes** Cook **25 minutes**

 FODMAP-Lite   **Freezer**

Inspired by the Greek spinach pie, spanakopita, that I love so much, this version packs in loads of veggies and flavor. It's an ideal centerpiece for lunch with friends and is a hit at picnics and for hungry kids. With 6 grams of fiber per portion, you won't mind when the kids come back for seconds.

1 cup (250 g) ricotta
7 ounces (200 g) feta, crumbled
⅔ cup (100 g) peas, fresh or frozen
3 ounces (85 g) green beans, diced
1 cup (10 g) dill, roughly chopped
1⅓ cups (40 g) spinach, finely chopped
5 cups (150 g) mixed greens,
    roughly chopped
6 phyllo sheets
1 tablespoon sesame seeds
Extra virgin olive oil, for brushing
Sea salt
Fresh ground black pepper

1. Preheat the oven to 425°F (220°C). Line a baking sheet with parchment paper.

2. Wilt the mixed greens and spinach—either in a large saucepan with a splash of water over medium heat or in the microwave for 3 minutes. Allow to cool, then, using clean hands, squeeze out any excess moisture and transfer to a large bowl.

3. Add the ricotta, feta, peas, beans, and dill, and mix well to combine. Season to taste.

4. Lay a phyllo sheet on your work surface (landscape). Brush a little oil down one short edge and attach another sheet. Repeat to make one long strip of 3 phyllo sheets. Brush oil all over the sheets and lay 3 additional sheets on top, to make 2 layers.

5. Spread the filling out in a long line down the edge closest to you, leaving a ¾-inch (2 cm) border. Then, start to tightly roll the sheets; keep rolling until you have one long tube. Brush the top with olive oil.

6. To make the swirl, take one end and gently roll it in on itself. Continue with the whole roll until you have a large spiral pie.

7. Transfer to the baking sheet and sprinkle with the sesame seeds. Bake in the oven for 25 to 30 minutes, until the phyllo is golden and crisp. Best eaten straight out of the oven.

Storage Leftovers can be kept in the fridge for up to 3 days. This pie can also be prepped in advance and kept in the freezer for up to 1 month—just add 5 to 10 minutes to the cooking time.

Tip Work quickly with the phyllo, otherwise it will dry out. Brush with oil if it becomes too dry to roll.

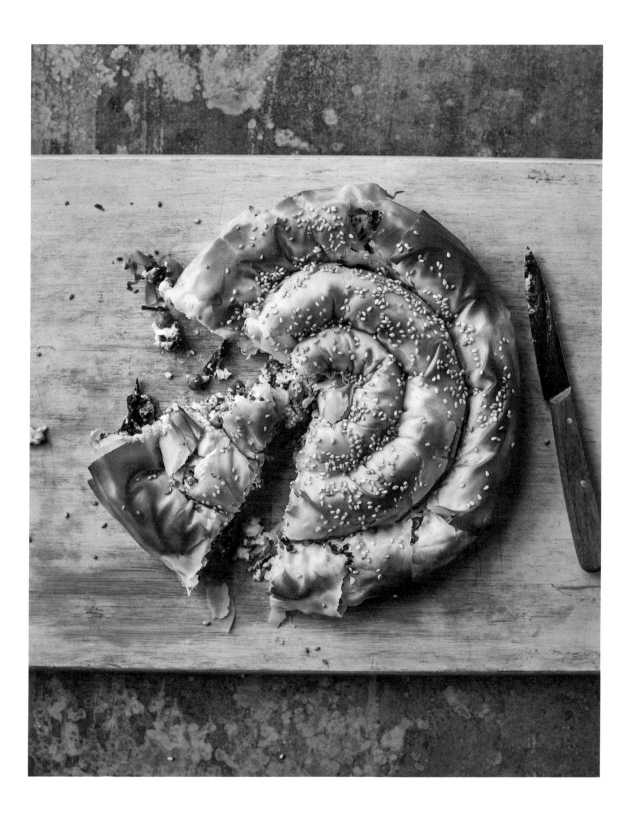

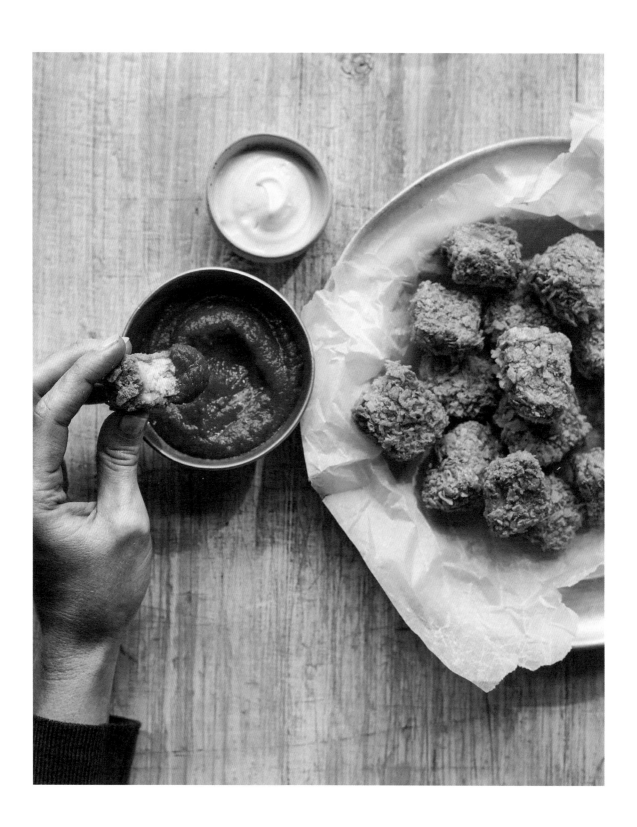

Popcorn Chick-less Nuggets

Plant Points
2.25

Makes **16 nuggets**   Prep **10 minutes**   Cook **15 minutes**

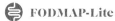 **FODMAP-Lite**

Are you a sucker for ultra-processed chicken nuggets? I used to be, too! But then I discovered these equally crispy and juicy plant-based alternatives. Take each mouthful to the next level with a dip of Garlicky Aquafaba Aioli (page 172) or No-Added-Sugar Ketchup (page 175).

10 ounces (280 g) extra-firm tofu

⅓ cup plus 1 tablespoon (95 ml) soy milk or milk of choice

⅓ cup (50 g) whole wheat flour or flour of choice

½ teaspoon smoked paprika

Pinch of sea salt

2 tablespoons nutritional yeast (optional)

¾ cup (75 g) corn flakes, crushed

1. Preheat the oven to 400°F (200°C). Line a baking sheet with parchment paper.

2. Cut the tofu into 1 x 1 x ¾-inch (3 x 3 x 2 cm) nuggets.

3. In a large bowl, mix the milk, flour, paprika, salt, and the nutritional yeast (if using). Stir to form a thick batter.

4. Place the crushed corn flakes in a separate bowl.

5. Dip each tofu nugget into the batter, shaking off any excess, before rolling it in the crushed corn flakes. Place on the baking sheet. Once all of the nuggets are coated, pop in the oven for 15 minutes or until golden and crispy. Best enjoyed straight out of the oven.

Switch Experiment with herbs and spices; instead of the paprika, try mixed herbs, cumin, or thyme.

Zucchini and Hazelnut Salad

Plant Points
9.5

Serves **2**   Prep **10 minutes**   Cook **5 minutes**

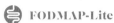 **FODMAP-Lite**

When you and your microbes are craving something light and refreshing that doesn't fall short on plant points or flavor, look no further. This light bite will really hit the spot, giving you 7 grams of fiber and getting you 9.5 plant points closer to your weekly target.

¼ cup (about 30 g) hazelnuts

3 tablespoons mixed seeds

2 zucchini

1⅓ cup (40 g) mixed salad greens
(e.g., spinach, arugula, watercress)

2 ounces (60 g) feta, crumbled

Dressing

1 tablespoon extra virgin olive oil

Juice of ½ orange (about 3 tablespoons),
plus zest to taste

2 teaspoons apple cider vinegar

1 teaspoon honey

Sea salt

Fresh ground black pepper

Toppings

2 teaspoons mint leaves, finely chopped

⅓ cup (50 g) pomegranate seeds

1. Preheat the oven to 350°F (180°C).

2. Spread the hazelnuts out on a baking sheet and bake for 5 minutes, until golden, adding the seeds to the tray for the final 2 minutes. Set aside to cool, then roughly chop the hazelnuts.

3. To make the dressing, mix the orange zest, orange juice, olive oil, vinegar, and honey in a small bowl. Season to taste.

4. Using a vegetable peeler, peel the zucchini into ribbons. Transfer to a small bowl, then pour the dressing on top. Allow to marinate for a few minutes before tossing in the greens.

5. Divide the mixture between two serving bowls, followed by the feta, hazelnuts, and seeds.

6. Pour over any leftover dressing before scattering the mint leaves and pomegranate seeds (if using) on top.

Note Want to turn this into a main meal? It goes perfectly with a grilled fillet of white fish and a side of toasted sourdough.

Leafy Taco Wraps

Serves **2**   Prep **10 minutes**

A flavor-filled bean mixture nestled in a crisp lettuce cup, this wrap is perfect for a light bite or lunch on the go—and it feeds your gut 16 grams of fiber, too (that's more than half your daily needs!). Want a heartier option to transform your Taco Tuesdays? Swap the lettuce for whole wheat tortillas.

1 ear fresh corn, or ⅔ cup (100 g) canned corn

One 15-ounce (425 g) can black-eyed peas, drained and rinsed

½ cup (100 g) fresh salsa

1 small avocado, diced

2 jarred roasted red peppers, roughly chopped

1 ounce (30 g) feta, chopped into ½-inch (1 cm) cubes

¼ teaspoon ground cumin

Sea salt

Fresh ground black pepper

4 large lettuce leaves

To Serve (optional)

3 tablespoons fresh cilantro

¼ cup (60 g) probiotic yogurt

1 fresh chile, sliced

½ lime, cut into wedges

1. Cut the corn off the cob and add to a large bowl. Add the black-eyed peas, salsa, avocado, red peppers, feta, and cumin. Toss to combine and season to taste.

2. To serve, lay out the lettuce leaves. Place a large spoonful of the bean mixture on each leaf, followed by the cilantro, yogurt, chile, and lime (if using).

3. Roll up the lettuce wraps and dig in.

Switch   Can't get your hands on black-eyed peas? Use canned black beans or kidney beans instead. You can also swap the roasted red pepper for fresh bell pepper.

Storage   The bean mixture will keep in the fridge for 3 days. See the Tip on page 173 to prevent the avocado from browning. But even if it does go brown, it's still perfectly good to eat!

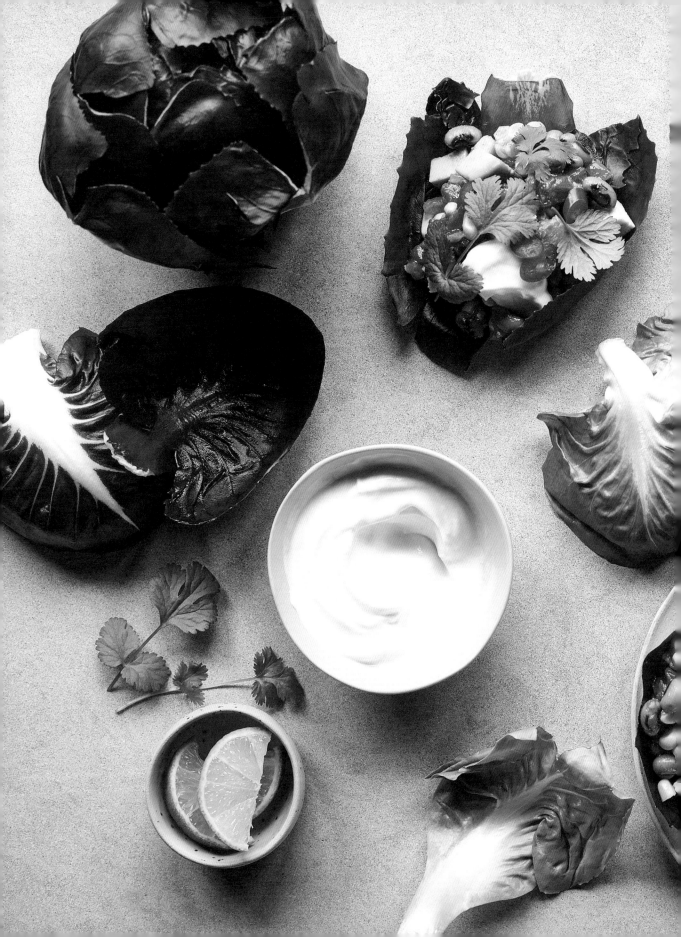

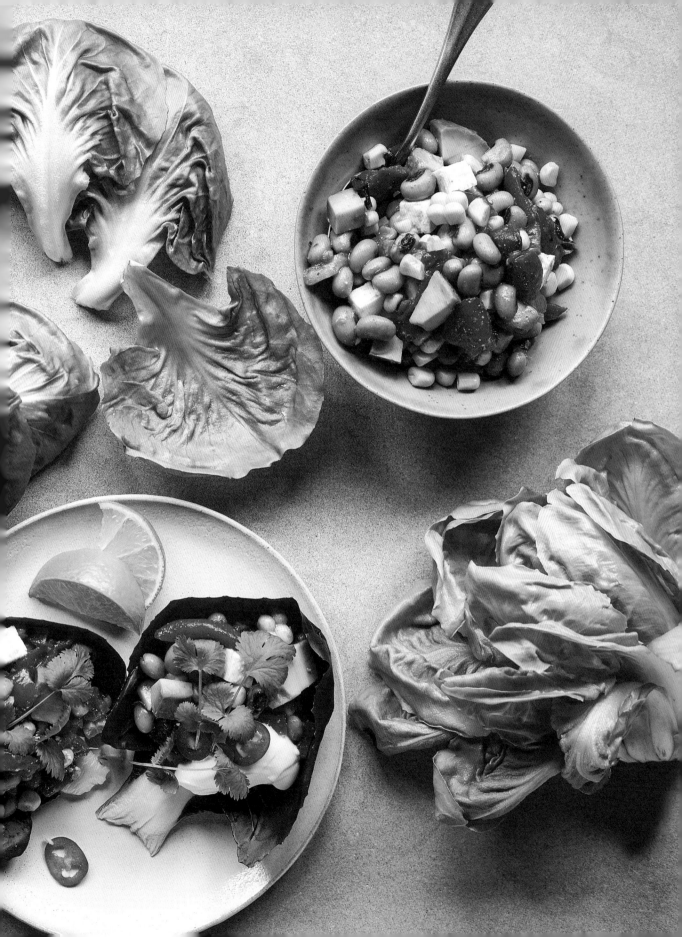

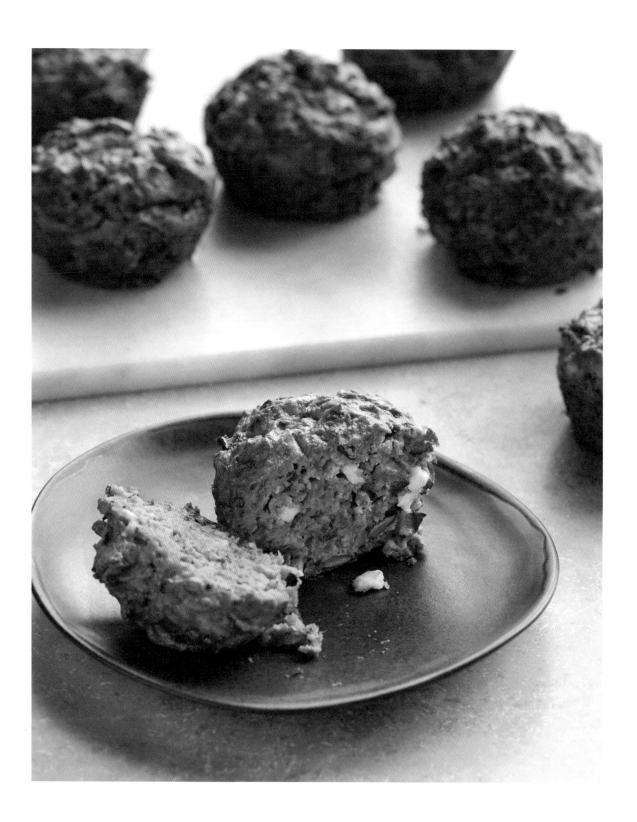

Butternut Muffins

Plant Points
7

Makes **12 muffins**   Prep **15 minutes**   Cook **30 minutes**

 FODMAP-Lite   **Freezer**

These savory, moist muffins are ideal to make in bulk and then freeze, so you always have something tasty and nourishing ready to go when hunger strikes. Great for lunch boxes or as an afternoon snack.

Olive oil, for greasing
10.5 ounces (300 g) butternut
    squash, grated
1 zucchini (about 5 ounces/140 g),
    grated
1⅓ cup (160 g) spelt flour or flour
    of choice
2 teaspoons baking powder
4 large eggs, beaten
3 tablespoons extra virgin olive oil
3.5 ounces (100 g) feta, crumbled
3 tablespoons mixed seeds
⅔ cup (10 g) fresh basil, finely chopped
2 teaspoons smoked paprika
1 teaspoon red pepper flakes (optional)
½ teaspoon sea salt, or to taste
Splash of milk of choice (optional)

1. Preheat the oven to 400°F (200°C). Grease a 12-cup muffin pan and add a disc of parchment paper to the bottom of each hole to prevent sticking.

2. Place the grated squash and zucchini in a large bowl. Add the flour and baking powder and stir to coat.

3. Add the eggs and the oil, and stir well to incorporate evenly.

4. Add the feta, seeds, basil, paprika, red pepper flakes (if using), and salt, and stir well to form a thick batter. If it's a little dry, add a splash of milk.

5. Fill each muffin cup to just below the top, allowing room for them to rise. Bake for 30 to 35 minutes, until a skewer comes out clean. Place on a wire rack to cool. Enjoy warm from the oven, or cold the next day.

Storage These muffins will keep in the fridge for 3 days in an airtight container. You can also freeze them for up to 2 months and defrost in the microwave when hunger strikes.

Tip For an extra plant point, add in ⅓ cup (50 g) of frozen peas.

Switch If squash isn't in season, use sweet potato instead.

Packed Lunches

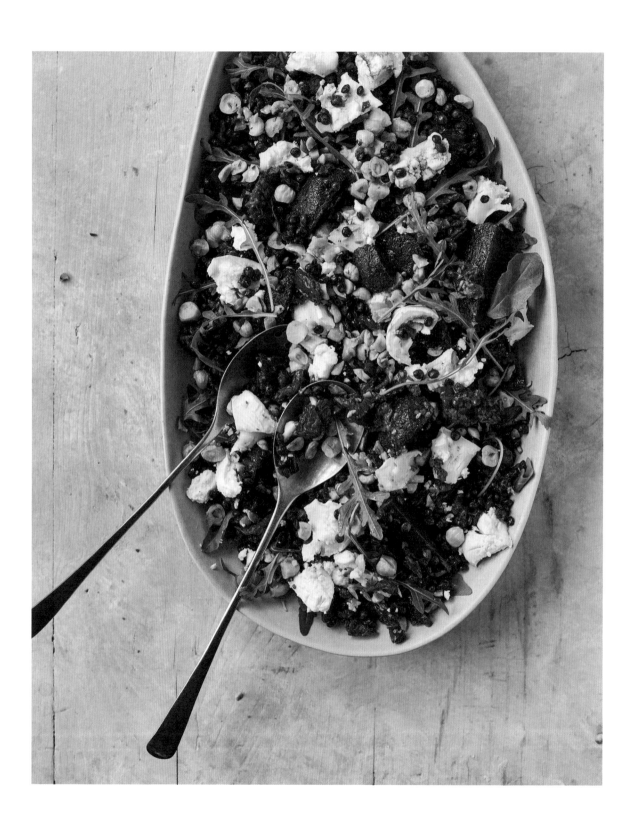

Beet, Lentil, and Goat Cheese Salad

Plant Points
5.25

Serves **4**   Prep **10 minutes**   Cook **5 minutes**

Boring salads have no place on my plate! This winning combo features layers of earthy flavors rounded off with creamy goat cheese and has a whopping 14 grams of fiber per portion. It might even have you making a double batch next time.

One 15-ounce (425 g) can Puy or
    green lentils
4 large cooked beets, cut into wedges
20 sun-dried tomato halves, preserved
    in oil, roughly chopped

Dressing
2 tablespoons balsamic vinegar
1 teaspoon honey or sweetener of choice
2 tablespoons extra virgin olive oil

Toppings
2 cups (60 g) salad greens
    (e.g., spinach, arugula, watercress)
5.5 ounces (160 g) goat cheese, crumbled
½ cup (65 g) hazelnuts

1. Add the lentils, beets, and sun-dried tomatoes to a large bowl.

2. In a small bowl, whisk together the vinegar, honey, and oil. Pour over the lentils and veggies. Let marinate for at least 5 minutes (ideally 30 minutes, if you have the time) while you prep the toppings.

3. Preheat the oven to 350°F (180°C).

4. Place the hazelnuts on a baking sheet and bake for 5 minutes until golden. Set aside to cool, then chop roughly.

5. For lunch on the go, add the marinated mixture to a glass jar, followed by the goat cheese, hazelnuts, and greens, to prevent them from getting soggy. Give it a good stir before digging in.

6. For a leisurely lunch, place the greens on a large serving tray, followed by the marinated mixture. Top with goat cheese and the hazelnuts. Toss before serving—yum!

Storage   The marinated mixture will keep for up to 3 days in the fridge. The salad also keeps in the fridge for up to 3 days, but the leaves are best added fresh as you serve to prevent them from getting soggy.

Roasted Veggie and Freekeh Salad

Plant Points
9.5

Serves **4**   Prep **10 minutes**   Cook **25 minutes**

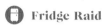 **Fridge Raid**

A hearty Middle Eastern–inspired salad, full of flavor and designed to keep you fiber-fueled past the 3 PM slump. I love a combination of peppers, zucchini, red onion, green beans, cherry tomatoes, cauliflower, and fresh corn, but any of your favorites or leftovers will work, too.

28 ounces (800 g) mixed vegetables (I love ready-to-roast, Mediterranean-style veggies), roughly chopped

2 tablespoons extra virgin olive oil

1 tablespoon harissa, or more to taste

1¼ cups (250 g) freekeh or whole grains of choice

2 tablespoons mixed seeds

¼ cup (25 g) pecans or nut of choice

1⅓ cup (40 g) salad greens

Sea salt

Fresh ground black pepper

To Serve (optional)

¼ cup (60 g) probiotic yogurt

2 teaspoons harissa

Fresh parsley

1. Preheat the oven to 400°F (200°C).

2. Place the vegetables in a large roasting pan. Stir the oil and harissa together before drizzling over the veggies and season to taste. Use your hands to mix everything together. Roast in the oven for 15 minutes.

3. Cook the freekeh according to package directions (about 20 minutes in boiling water). Set aside to cool.

4. Remove the pan from the oven and turn the veggies. Scatter the mixed seeds and pecans on top and then return to the oven for another 10 minutes, or until golden brown.

5. Add the cooled freekeh to a large bowl along with the salad greens and the roasted veggies, and toss to combine.

6. Combine the yogurt and harissa (if using), then dollop on top of the veggies. Sprinkle with parsley.

Tip Any time you're having roasted vegetables, make a double batch to use for this dish.

Smoked Mackerel, New Potato, and Apple Salad

Plant Points
8.5

Serves **4**   Prep **10 minutes**   Cook **15 minutes**

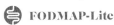 **FODMAP-Lite**

Don't be deceived by its simplicity—this salad oozes flavor. Delicious warm or cold, there's something extra-special about the delicate smoked fish, crunchy apple, and tender veggies, wrapped in a creamy dressing with a subtle tang from the mustard. It's also a good source of fiber, including resistant starch from the chilled potatoes, and omega-3.

12 baby new potatoes, halved
8 ounces (225 g) asparagus
    spears, trimmed
½ cup (65 g) cashews
2 apples, cored and sliced
2 fennel bulbs, sliced
11 ounces (320 g) smoked mackerel
2⅔ cups (80 g) mixed greens
Sea salt

Dressing
¼ cup (60 g) probiotic yogurt
2 teaspoons Dijon mustard
Juice of 1 lemon (about 3 tablespoons)
½ to 1 cup (5 to 10 g) fresh dill,
    chopped, to taste
Fresh ground black pepper

1. Preheat the oven to 350°F (180°C).

2. Fill a medium saucepan with water, then add the potatoes along with a pinch of salt. Boil for 15 minutes or until tender.

3. Add the asparagus spears to the potatoes for the last 3 minutes of cooking, then drain everything and set aside to cool slightly.

4. While the potatoes are cooking, place the cashews on a baking sheet and bake for 5 minutes or until golden. Remove from the oven and set aside to cool.

5. To make the dressing, whisk together the yogurt, mustard, lemon juice, dill, and pepper in a large bowl. Add the potatoes, asparagus, cashews, apple, fennel, and mackerel and stir to combine.

6. When ready to serve, toss in the greens and season to taste.

Switch Not into mackerel? Switch it out for your fish of choice, an egg, or legumes, such as butter beans.

Storage This will keep in the fridge for up to 3 days, but the greens are best added fresh as you serve to prevent them from wilting.

Baked Sweet Potato Trio

Don't underestimate the versatility of sweet potato. Creamy flavor aside, they're also a nourishing source of fiber and are loaded with beta-carotene, one of those phytochemicals with impressive antioxidant powers. Plus, the toppings deliver at least a third of your daily fiber needs, too. Sweet, savory, hot or cold—this trio can flex around your mood.

Baked Sweet Potato with Black Beans

Plant Points
5.25

Serves **2**   Prep **5 minutes**   Cook **50 minutes**

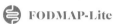 FODMAP-Lite

2 sweet potatoes (about 6 ounces/180 g each)

1½ tablespoon extra virgin olive oil

1 garlic clove, grated or crushed

One 15-ounce (425 g) can black beans, drained and rinsed

2⅔ cups (80 g) fresh spinach

¼ teaspoon cayenne

Sea salt

Fresh ground black pepper

2 tablespoons probiotic yogurt

½ avocado, sliced (about 3 ounces/80 g)

2 pickled jalapeños

Fresh cilantro

Lime wedges (optional)

1. To bake the sweet potatoes, prick them with a fork (to prevent the skin from splitting). Cook either in the microwave with a splash of water for 8 to 10 minutes, until tender all the way through, or in the oven for 50 minutes at 400°F (200°C).

2. While the potatoes are cooking, make the filling. Heat the olive oil in a saucepan over medium heat and add the garlic. Cook for 1 minute. Add the beans and cook for a few more minutes to heat all the way through before stirring in the spinach and cayenne. Cover for 2 minutes to wilt the spinach, then stir. Taste and adjust the cayenne, and season to taste.

3. Cut each sweet potato in half and fill with the bean mixture. Top with the yogurt, avocado, 1 jalapeño, some cilantro, and a squeeze of lime juice (if using). Season to taste.

Storage   This will keep in the fridge for up to 3 days.

Switch   Already had black beans this week? Switch them out for pinto beans.

Tip   Cook extra sweet potato to make the One-Minute Sweet Potato Slider on page 304.

Baked Sweet Potato with Nut-Free Pesto

Serves **2**   Prep **15 minutes**   Cook **50 minutes**

 FODMAP-Lite   **Freezer**

2 sweet potatoes
1 teaspoon extra virgin olive oil
One 15-ounce (425 g) can butter
    beans, drained and rinsed
1 teaspoon za'atar
Sea salt
Fresh ground black pepper

Pesto
¼ cup (60 ml) extra virgin olive oil
1.5 ounces (40 g) Parmesan, grated
¼ cup (40 g) pumpkin seeds, toasted
2 cups (30 g) fresh basil, plus more
    to serve
Juice of ½ lemon (about
    1½ tablespoons)
1 small garlic clove
Sea salt
Fresh ground black pepper

Cherry tomatoes, halved

1. Cook the sweet potatoes following the instructions on the previous page.

2. Heat the oil in a medium frying pan over medium heat. Add the beans and za'atar and cook for a few more minutes to heat the beans all the way through. Remove from the heat and season to taste.

3. To make the pesto, place the oil, Parmesan, pumpkin seeds, basil, lemon juice, and garlic in a food processor and pulse until you have a textured green paste. Season to taste.

4. Cut the potatoes in half and top with the butter bean mixture, pesto, tomatoes, and a few basil leaves.

Storage Any leftover pesto can be kept in fridge for up to 1 week. Cover the surface with either a drizzle of olive oil or plastic wrap to keep it fresh and green. You can also freeze it for up to 3 months.

PB & J Baked Sweet Potato

Serves **2**   Prep **10 minutes**   Cook **50 minutes**

 FODMAP-Lite   **Freezer**

2 sweet potatoes

Chia-Berry Jam
1½ cups (250 g) frozen raspberries
Juice of ½ orange (about
    3 tablespoons)
2 tablespoons chia seeds
Honey or sweetener of choice, to taste

1 banana, sliced
Sprinkle of cinnamon
2 tablespoons nut butter of choice
2 teaspoons coconut flakes or mixed
    seeds, toasted (optional)

1. Cook the sweet potatoes following the instructions on the previous page.

2. To make the jam, place the raspberries and orange juice in a small saucepan over medium heat and simmer for 5 to 7 minutes, until the berries have broken down and the liquid has reduced. Remove from the heat, stir in the seeds, and let stand for a few minutes until thickened. Sweeten to taste.

3. While the jam thickens, sprinkle the banana with cinnamon. Heat a small frying pan over medium heat. Add the banana and cook for 30 seconds on each side or until caramelized.

4. Cut the potatoes in half and add the banana, 2 tablespoons of jam per potato, a drizzle of nut butter, and coconut or seeds (if using).

Storage The jam will keep in the fridge for up to 1 week in an airtight container. It can be frozen for up to 3 months.

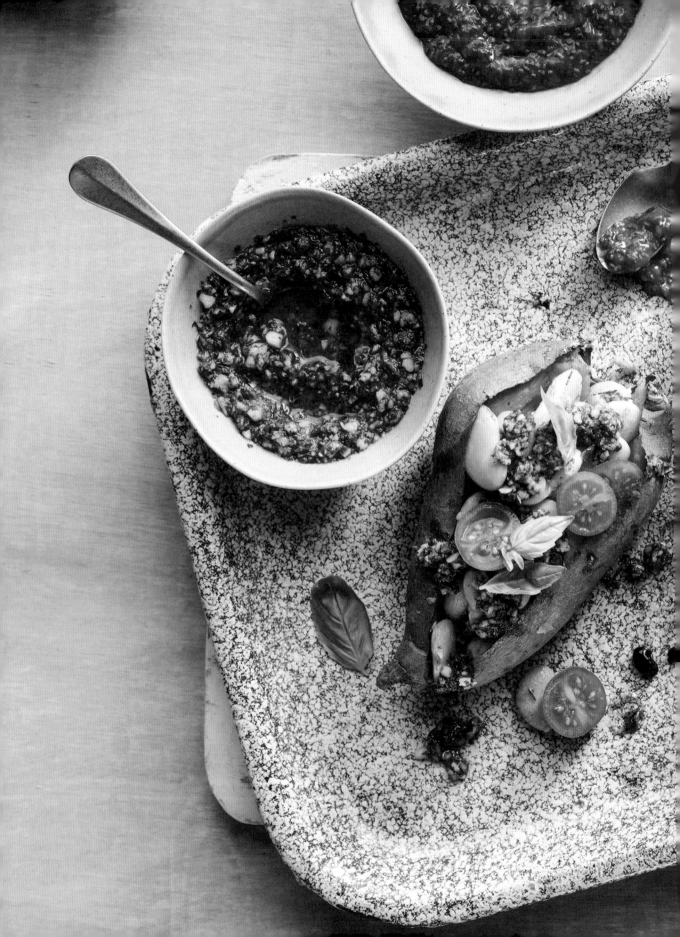

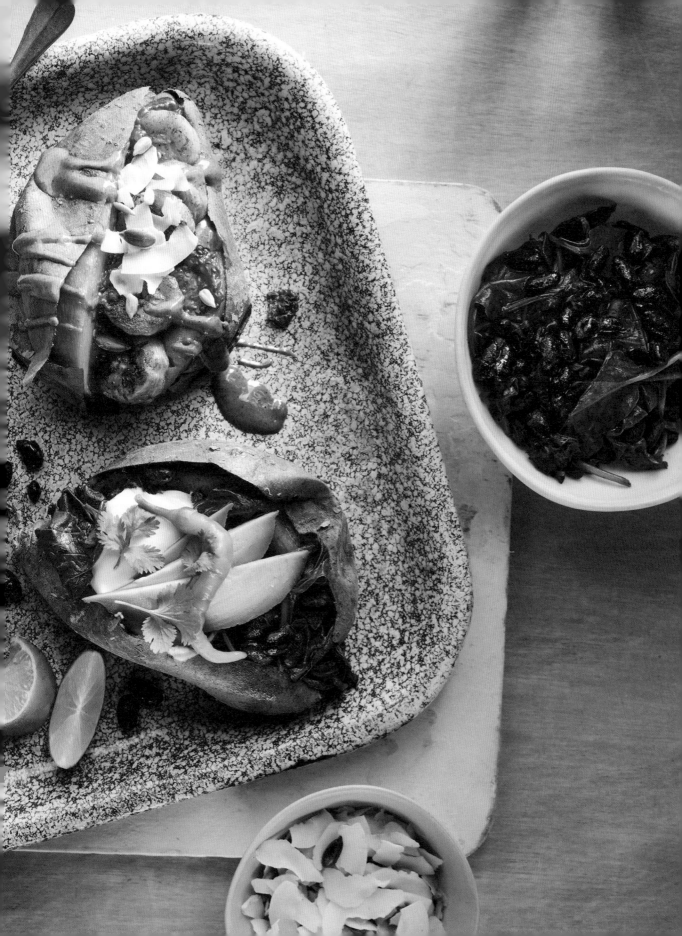

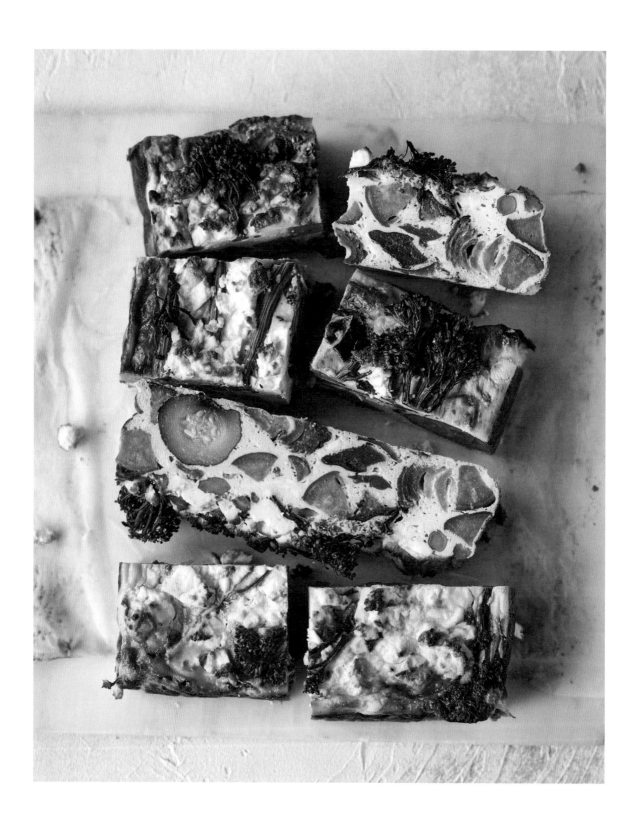

Chunky Veggie and Feta Frittata

Plant Points
6.75

Serves **8** Prep **15 minutes** Cook **1 hour 20 minutes**

 FODMAP-Lite   **Fridge Raid**

Hot or cold, for breakfast, lunch, or dinner—things don't get much more versatile than this fiber-filled frittata. Mix up the veggies to keep it seasonal and interesting for endless weekday options. It's earned a regular spot on my menu.

1 red onion (about 6 ounces/170 g), cut into 8 wedges

1 zucchini (about 7 ounces/200 g), cut into 4 long quarters

1 eggplant (about 14 ounces/400 g), cut into 8 long strips

1 red bell pepper (about 5 ounces/ 140 g), cut into 6 long strips

2 sweet potatoes (about 10.5 ounces/300 g), each cut into 6 long strips

4 thyme sprigs, leaves picked, or 1 teaspoon dried thyme

2 teaspoons red pepper flakes (optional)

10 large eggs

¼ cup (60 ml) extra virgin olive oil, plus more for drizzling

Generous ¾ cup (200 g) full-fat Greek yogurt

8 Broccolini stalks

7 ounces (200 g) feta, crumbled

1. Preheat the oven to 400°F (200°C).

2. Line a large baking sheet with parchment paper. Place the eggplant, sweet potatoes, zucchini, onion, and bell pepper onto the baking sheet. Mix with the thyme leaves, a generous drizzle of olive oil, a big pinch of salt, and red pepper flakes (if using). Roast for 30 minutes until softened.

3. Line the base and sides of a deep 10-inch (25 cm) square baking pan. Layer the roasted veggies into the pan, alternating the different types. This will ensure that each slice of frittata has a selection of veggies when cut.

4. Stir together the eggs, olive oil, and yogurt until just combined, along with a big pinch of salt and a grind of pepper. Pour this mix over the veggies, then add the Broccolini and sprinkle the feta on top.

5. Reduce oven temperature to 350°F (180°C). Bake for 50 to 60 minutes, until the middle has just set. If the top starts to brown earlier, cover with foil.

6. When the frittata is done, the center should no longer jiggle. For extra reassurance, cut into the center. If raw egg runs into the cut, it needs a little more time in the oven.

7. Let cool for at least 10 minutes, then slice to serve.

Tip You can use probiotic yogurt instead of full-fat Greek here—the microbes die off in high temperatures, so there's no extra benefit to using it in this recipe, but there's also no downside!

Storage This will keep in the fridge for up to 3 days.

Tofu Fried Whole Grains with Crunchy Cashews

Plant Points 12.5

Serves **2**   Prep **15 minutes**   Cook **10 minutes (or 25 minutes if cooking whole grains)**

 FODMAP-Lite   **Fridge Raid**

It's easy to get stuck in a whole-grain rut, eating the same types on repeat. This deliciously diverse take on fried rice is here to show you that there are so many amazing textures and flavors in the world of whole grains. Plus, it doesn't just deliver on flavor, but fiber (11 grams) and plant points (12.5), too, delivering a third of your daily and weekly goals respectively.

9 ounces (255 g) precooked mixed whole grains, or 3.5 ounces (100 g) raw whole grains
⅓ cup (45 g) cashews
2 teaspoons sesame oil
1 large red chile, finely chopped (optional)
2 garlic cloves, grated or minced
2 teaspoons peeled, grated fresh ginger
3 cups (200 g) mixed sliced stir-fry vegetables (e.g., cabbage, carrots, peppers, red onion)
½ cup (50 g) bean sprouts (optional)
⅓ cup (50 g) peas, fresh or frozen
1 scallion, sliced
1 tablespoon soy sauce, plus more to taste
Sea salt
Fresh ground black pepper

Tofu Scramble
1 teaspoon sesame oil
5 ounces (150 g) silken tofu
1 tablespoon nutritional yeast (optional)
¼ teaspoon paprika
¼ teaspoon ground turmeric
¼ teaspoon black pepper

1. If you're cooking your own whole grains, cook them according to the package instructions.

2. Heat a large frying pan over medium heat. Add the cashews and toast for a few minutes, stirring frequently. Remove from the pan and set aside.

3. To make the tofu scramble, heat 1 teaspoon sesame oil in the same pan. Crumble in the tofu with your hands, then add the nutritional yeast (if using), paprika, turmeric, and black pepper. Cook until any liquid has reduced, 3 to 4 minutes. Remove from the pan and set aside.

4. To the same pan, add another teaspoon of sesame oil along with the chile (if using), garlic, and ginger, and cook for 1 minute. Add the stir-fry vegetables, bean sprouts (if using), and peas. Cook for 3 to 4 minutes, so the veggies still have a little crunch to them.

5. Stir in the tofu scramble, whole grains, scallion, and soy sauce, and cook for 1 to 2 minutes to heat through.

6. Taste and adjust seasoning to preference, then serve topped with the toasted cashews.

Tip You can always switch out the tofu scramble for two large eggs, scrambled, with turmeric and black pepper.

Storage This will keep in the fridge for up to 3 days.

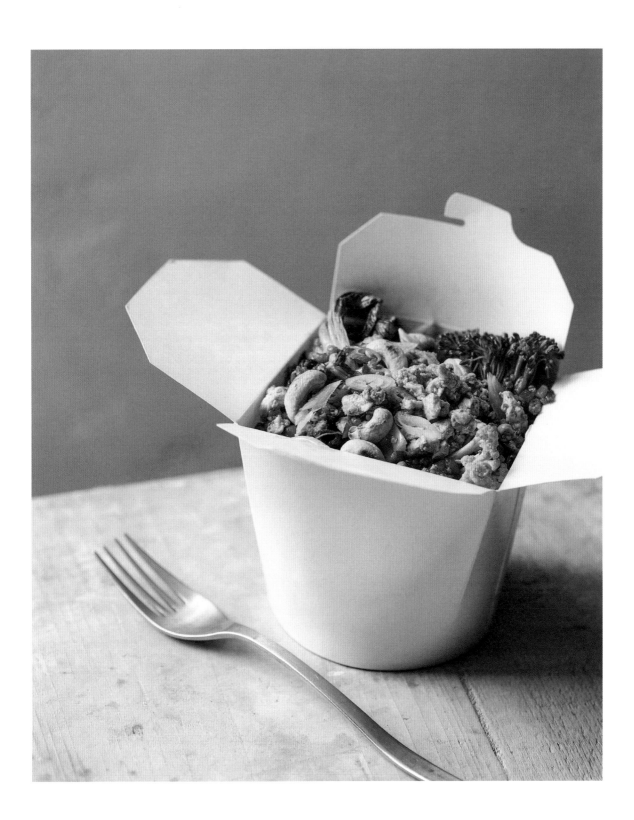

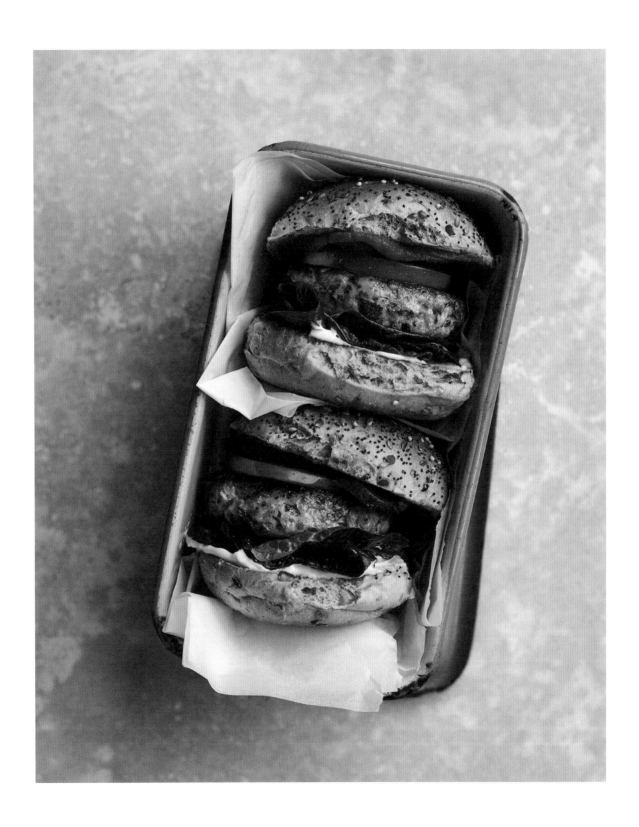

Reinvented Chicken Burgers

Plant Points
4

Serves **2**   Prep **5 minutes**   Cook **10 minutes**

FODMAP-Lite   ✳ **Freezer**

Left overnight for the flavors to really infuse, this burger mix is even better the second time around. Pair with crispy lettuce, juicy tomato, and beets, and top with a dollop of creamy aioli and ketchup for the ultimate burger. You can add any other toppings you like: Some of my favorites are grilled onions, a fried egg, avocado, or portobello mushrooms.

1½ teaspoons extra virgin olive oil
1 cup (230 g) Chicken 'n' Veggie
   Meatball mix (see page 258)

To Serve
2 seedy burger buns
2 large lettuce leaves
1 large tomato, sliced
4 slices pickled beet
Garlicky Aquafaba Aioli (page 172)
No-Sugar-Added Ketchup (page 175)

1. Divide the chicken mixture in half and with clean hands, make two burgers.

2. Heat the olive oil in a frying pan over medium-high heat, and cook the burgers until golden brown on the outside and cooked through, 5 to 6 minutes.

3. Slice the burger buns (you can also toast them if you like), then layer up the lettuce, tomato, beet, aioli, and ketchup to make a classic burger and enjoy!

Storage The cooked burgers can be frozen for up to 1 month.

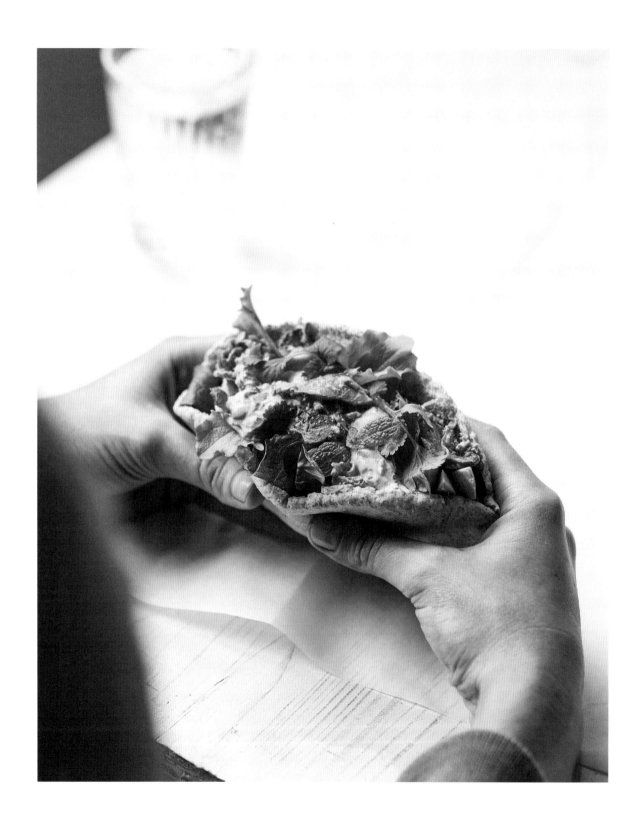

Reinvented Saucy Mushroom Pita Pockets

Serves **1**   Prep **10 minutes**

Pitas are perfect for stuffing in those plant points—literally! These are a great way to have a satisfying and gut-loving lunch on the run using the leftover saucy mushrooms from my phyllo parcels (page 224). It also provides almost a third of your daily fiber needs.

1 whole wheat pita (or wrap)

⅓ cup (80 g) leftover Saucy Mushrooms (see Phyllo Parcels with Saucy Mushrooms, page 224), or as much as you can get in

½ avocado, sliced (about 2.5 ounces/70 g)

½ red bell pepper, sliced

⅔ cup (20 g) mixed greens

1 tablespoon probiotic yogurt

½ teaspoon harissa (optional)

Fresh herbs (e.g., mint and cilantro)

1. Toast the pita until warm and slice in half. Split it open and stuff with the mushrooms, avocado, bell pepper, and mixed greens. If you prefer your saucy mushrooms warm, heat them in the microwave for a minute or two before adding to your pita.

2. Mix the yogurt with the harissa (if using), then dollop on top of the stuffing with as many fresh herbs as you like.

Switch If you don't have any peppers handy, this works well with sliced radish, scallions, or cherry tomatoes.

Storage These are best eaten the same day.

Reinvented Couscous Salad

Serves **2**   Prep **10 minutes**

Cook once, eat twice. This simple recipe shows how easy it is to turn leftover roasted vegetables (like the veggies in the Rainbow Roast with Green Yorkshire Puddings on page 253) into a whole new meal. The flavorsome combo of spices does all the heavy lifting; you just need to chop, pour, and combine.

Heaping 1 cup (200 g) couscous

1 teaspoon ras el hanout (or 1 teaspoon ground cumin and ½ teaspoon ground cinnamon)

¼ teaspoon ground turmeric

1 cup (240 ml) vegetable stock, hot

2 tablespoons extra virgin olive oil

One 15-ounce (425 g) can chickpeas, drained and rinsed

10 to 14 ounces (300 to 400 g) leftover vegetables (see Headnote), diced

⅔ cup (100 g) cherry tomatoes, chopped (optional)

10 dried apricots, chopped (about 2 ounces/60 g)

¼ cup (35 g) almonds, chopped (optional)

⅓ cup (50 g) raisins

½ cup (15 g) chopped fresh cilantro

Sea salt

Fresh ground black pepper

¼ cup (60 g) probiotic yogurt (optional)

1. Place the couscous in a large bowl, along with the ras el hanout and turmeric. Pour over the hot stock and olive oil and stir to combine. Cover the bowl with an upturned plate for 5 minutes, then use a fork to fluff up the grains.

2. Add the chickpeas, roasted vegetables, tomatoes (if using), apricots, almonds (if using), raisins, and cilantro, season to taste and mix to combine. Top with yogurt (if using) before digging in.

Switch Not a fan of raisins? Switch for goji berries.

Storage This will keep in the fridge for 2 days.

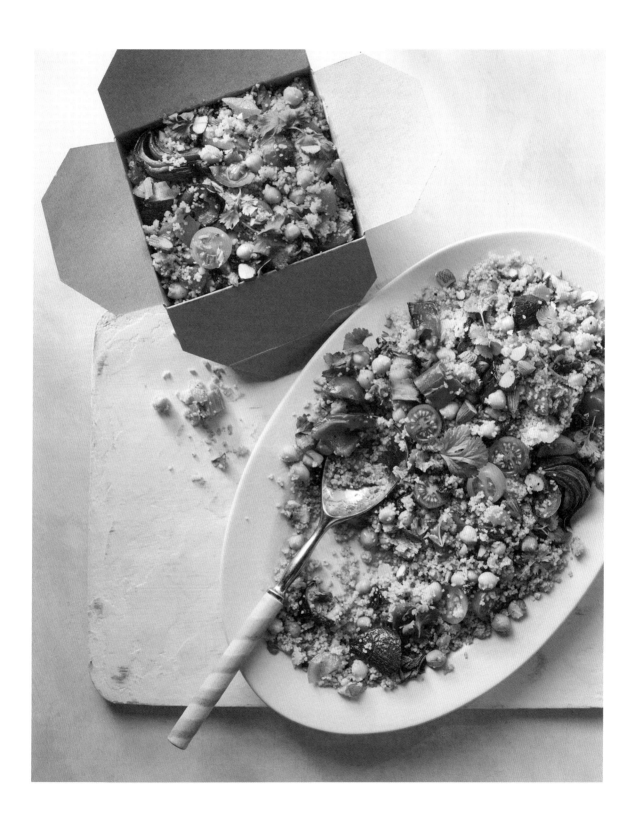

Thai-Inspired Fish Cakes and Crunchy Salad

Serves **2**   Prep **10 minutes**   Cook **10 minutes**

 FODMAP-Lite   **Freezer**

Because plant-based doesn't mean *only* plants. This dish celebrates the gut-loving omega-3-filled salmon and is packed full of plant flavors and colors. You'll want to make a double batch of these to fill your freezer.

Fish Cakes
1 large egg
3 scallions, roughly chopped
½ to 1 red chile, roughly chopped
1 fresh lemongrass stalk, roughly chopped or 2 teaspoons lemongrass paste
⅓ cup (10 g) chopped fresh cilantro
2 tablespoons unsweetened shredded coconut
1½ tablespoons peeled, roughly chopped fresh ginger
1½ teaspoons extra virgin olive oil
Sea salt
Fresh ground black pepper
One 6-ounce (175 g) can pink or red salmon or fish of choice
Sesame oil, for frying

Salad
One 5-ounce (150 g) bag salad mix (or 1 cup/40 g watercress or leaves of choice, ½ cup (50 g) shredded carrot, 1 cup/70 g shredded cabbage)
⅓ cup (5 g) mixed fresh herbs of choice (cilantro, Thai basil, mint)

Dressing
Juice of 1 lime (about 2 tablespoons)
1 tablespoon soy sauce
1 teaspoon honey
½ teaspoon peeled, grated fresh ginger
Pinch of red pepper flakes (optional)

Chili sauce, for serving (optional)

1. To make the fish cakes, place the egg, scallions, chile, lemongrass, cilantro, coconut, ginger, and olive oil in a food processor and pulse until you have a fairly smooth mixture. Scrape down the sides a few times and pulse again to make sure it's all incorporated. Add a pinch of salt and pepper before forking in the fish.

2. Heat some sesame oil in a frying pan over medium-low heat. Using wet hands, form the mixture into four equal fish cakes and place in the pan. Fry gently with the lid on, until cooked through and golden brown, 4 to 5 minutes on each side.

3. While the fish cakes are cooking, make the salad. Place the salad mix and herbs in a large bowl. Make the dressing by combining the lime juice, soy sauce, honey, ginger, and red pepper flakes (if using) in a small bowl. Pour the dressing over the salad.

4. Serve the fish cakes with the salad and chili sauce (if using).

Storage The cooked fish cakes will keep for 3 days in the fridge. Or you can freeze them (cooked) for up to 1 month; defrost and reheat in the microwave or oven. The salad dressing will keep for 1 week in the fridge.

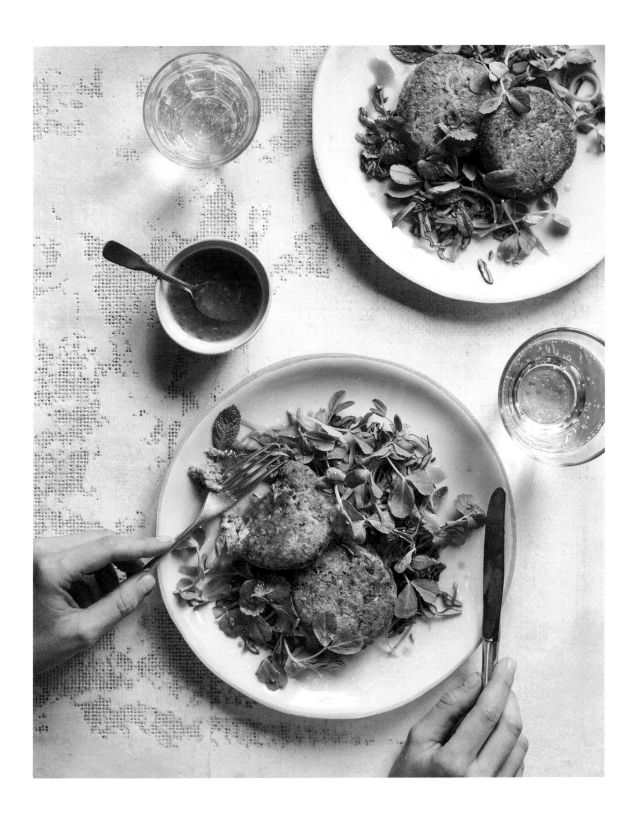

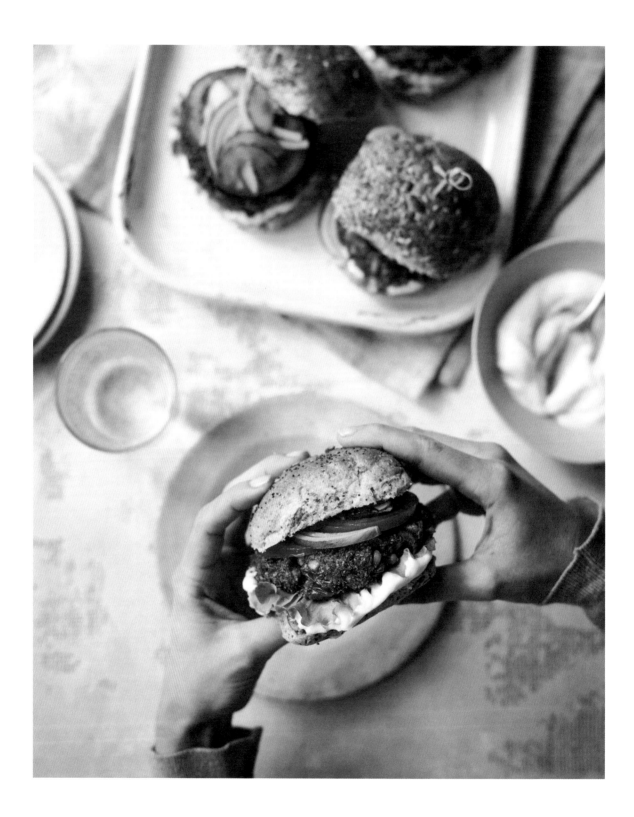

Smoky Beet Burger

Plant Points
10

Serves **6**   Prep **20 minutes**   Cook **10 minutes**

 Freezer

I like to think this is a pretty convincing alternative to a beef burger, with a delicious and nutritious twist. The smoky flavor and juicy texture of this burger, packed with 10 plant points, is guaranteed to make this a favorite in any meat-loving household. Each burger offers your microbes three times more fiber than your standard burger!

Quick Pickles (optional)
1 red onion, sliced
½ cucumber, sliced
3 tablespoons apple cider vinegar
1½ teaspoons sea salt
1 tablespoon coriander seeds

½ cup (50 g) flaxseed meal
3 tablespoons boiling water
⅔ cup (105 g) pine nuts,
    roughly chopped
Extra virgin olive oil, for frying
1 leek (about 3.5 ounces/100 g),
    finely chopped
2 garlic cloves, grated or chopped
2 cooked beets (about 7 ounces/
    200 g)
3 ounces (90 g) feta
½ cup (90 g) cooked quinoa
6 sun-dried tomato halves, preserved
    in oil, finely chopped
2 teaspoons arrowroot powder
    or cornstarch
2 teaspoons smoked paprika
Sea salt
Fresh ground black pepper

To Serve
6 whole wheat seedy buns
Garlicky Aquafaba Aioli (page 172)
3 tomatoes
6 large lettuce leaves

Storage These can be made ahead of time and refrigerated for up to 3 days. They can also be frozen, raw, for up to 1 month.

1. To make the pickles, place the onion, cucumber, vinegar, salt, and coriander seeds in a heatproof bowl with just enough boiling water to cover. Set aside.

2. To make the burgers, combine the flaxseed meal and boiling water in a small bowl. Set aside to allow it to thicken.

3. Meanwhile, in a frying pan, toast the pine nuts for 2 minutes. Transfer to a plate and set aside.

4. Heat some oil in the same frying pan over medium heat and cook the leek and garlic for a few minutes, until starting to brown.

5. Grate the beets into a large bowl. Squeeze out any excess liquid using a strainer.

6. Add the fried leek and garlic, feta, quinoa, pine nuts, flaxseed meal, sun-dried tomatoes, arrowroot powder, and smoked paprika. Use your hands to mix everything together (a pair of kitchen gloves comes in handy here, to stop your hands from becoming stained). Taste and season to preference. Using clean, wet hands, form the mixture into six equal patties, squeezing tightly together as you shape. If they feel too soft, sprinkle in some extra flaxseed.

7. Heat a thin layer of oil in the frying pan over medium-low heat, then add the burgers. Cook for 5 minutes with the lid on, then gently flip the burgers, and cook until lightly browned, 5 more minutes.

8. Transfer the patties to buns, add aioli, tomatoes, lettuce, and pickles (if desired).

Weeknight Dinners

Stir-Fry Adventures

Serves **2** Prep **5 minutes** Cook **5 to 10 minutes**

 FODMAP-Lite   **Fridge Raid**

Don't underestimate the power of a stir-fry when it comes to reaching your plant-point goals during those time-poor weeks—they're a staple on my menu. Although stir-frying is traditionally a Chinese technique, I've put together a stir-fry guide to show just how easy it is to fuse different flavors from other cultures to create a week's worth of diverse, tasty, and quick stir-fry dishes.

Choose one cuisine flavor, one protein, one whole grain, and one vegetable from the list below. Then follow the methods under your cuisine of choice for the ultimate stir-fry adventure.

Cuisine Flavor
- Indian
- Indonesian
- Italian
- Korean
- Thai

Protein
(about 6 ounces/180 g)
- Butter beans
- Cannellini beans
- Lentils
- Pinto beans
- Tofu

Whole Grain
(about 7 ounces/200 g)
- Barley
- Buckwheat noodles
- Mixed whole grains
- Rice noodles
- Sourdough bread

Vegetables
(about 10 ounces/300 g)
- Beans sprouts
- Bok choy
- Cabbage
- Corn
- Mushrooms
- Onions
- Peppers

Indian-Inspired Stir-Fry

Serves **2** Prep **5 minutes** Cook **10 minutes**

 FODMAP-Lite   **Fridge Raid**

Cuisine Flavor Base
1½ tablespoons extra virgin olive oil
2 garlic cloves, grated or crushed
2 teaspoons peeled, grated
   fresh ginger
1 teaspoon ground coriander
1 teaspoon ground cumin
¼ teaspoon ground turmeric
Sea salt
Fresh ground black pepper

Additional Vegetable (optional)
½ small cauliflower (about
   3.5 ounces/100 g),
   roughly chopped

To Serve
¼ cup (35 g) almonds, chopped
3 tablespoons fresh cilantro
½ teaspoon red pepper flakes

1. To make the cuisine flavor base, heat the olive oil in a medium frying pan or wok over medium heat. Add the garlic, ginger, coriander, cumin, and turmeric along with the cauliflower (if using). Cook until the veggies start to soften, 3 to 4 minutes, adding a splash of water if the mixture starts to stick.

2. Add the stir-fry veggies and cook until the veggies are just cooked, with a little crunch to them, 5 minutes. Stir in your protein and whole grains of choice and cook until warmed through, 2 minutes. Taste and adjust seasoning.

3. Serve with almonds, cilantro, and red pepper flakes.

Note This stir-fry pairs well with cooked lentils and your rice of choice.

Storage This will keep in the fridge for up to 3 days.

Indonesian-Inspired Stir-Fry

Plant Points
10

Serves **2**   Prep **10 minutes**   Cook **5 minutes**

 FODMAP-Lite   **Fridge Raid**

Cuisine Flavor Base
2 shallots, finely chopped
1 lemongrass stalk, roughly chopped, or
    1 teaspoon lemongrass paste
1½ tablespoons peeled, roughly chopped
    fresh ginger (optional)
⅔ cup (160 ml) coconut cream
Juice of 1 lime (about 1½ tablespoons)
1 tablespoon soy sauce
½ teaspoon ground turmeric (optional)
3 tablespoons crunchy peanut butter
Sesame oil, for frying

Additional Vegetables (optional)
2 ounces (55 g) baby corn
2 ounces (55 g) green beans

To Serve
1 tablespoon roasted peanuts, chopped
1 teaspoon red pepper flakes

1. To make the cuisine flavor base, place the shallots, lemongrass, ginger, coconut cream, lime juice, soy sauce, and turmeric in a high-powered blender and blend until smooth, 1 to 2 minutes. Stir in the peanut butter.

2. Heat the sesame oil in a medium frying pan or wok over medium heat, along with the stir-fry vegetables (and additional vegetables, if using) and mix. Cook until the veggies are just cooked, with a little crunch to them, 5 minutes. In the final few minutes, stir in half the cuisine flavor base mixture along with your protein and whole grains of choice.

3. Stir through the remaining cuisine flavor base mixture gradually until you're happy with the consistency and flavor. Scatter the peanuts and red pepper flakes on top to serve.

Note This stir-fry works well with tofu (or cooked chicken or turkey) and buckwheat noodles.

Storage Any leftover sauce keeps in the fridge for up to 1 week. The stir-fry keeps in the fridge for up to 3 days.

Italian-Inspired Stir-Fry

Plant Points
8

Serves **2**   Prep **5 minutes**   Cook **5 minutes**

 FODMAP-Lite   **Fridge Raid**

Cuisine Flavor Base
3 tablespoons extra virgin olive oil
2 garlic cloves, grated or crushed
1 teaspoon small capers,
    roughly chopped
1 tablespoon Italian seasoning
1 ounce (30 g) Parmesan, grated, or
    1½ tablespoon nutritional yeast
Juice of ½ lemon (about
    1½ tablespoons), plus zest to taste

Additional Vegetables (optional)
⅔ cup (100 g) cherry
    tomatoes, halved

To Serve
2 tablespoons pine nuts

1. To make the cuisine flavor base, heat the oil in a medium frying pan or wok over medium heat. Add the garlic, capers, and Italian seasoning, along with the stir-fry vegetables and cook until softened, 5 minutes. In the final 2 minutes, stir in the cherry tomatoes (if using), Parmesan, lemon juice, and your protein of choice.

2. Scatter the pine nuts on top and serve with your whole grain of choice.

Note This stir-fry works well with Broccolini, cannellini or pinto beans, and sourdough bread on the side.

Korean-Inspired Stir-Fry

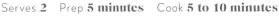

Plant Points 7.25

Serves **2** Prep **5 minutes** Cook **5 to 10 minutes**

 FODMAP-Lite   **Fridge Raid**

Cuisine Flavor Base
1½ tablespoons sesame oil
1½ tablespoons gochujang
   or sriracha
1 tablespoon mirin (optional)
1 tablespoon soy sauce
¼ teaspoon red pepper flakes
   (optional)

**Additional Vegetables
(optional)**
½ eggplant, sliced into
   ½-inch (1 cm) strips
2 tablespoons extra virgin
   olive oil

To Serve (optional)
1 tablespoon black or white
   sesame seeds

1. To make the cuisine flavor base, heat the sesame oil in a medium frying pan or wok over medium heat. Add the gochujang, mirin (if using), soy sauce, and red pepper flakes (if using), along with the eggplant and olive oil (if using) and cook until the eggplant is softened, 5 minutes. (If not using the eggplant, add the stir-fry vegetables right away.)

2. Add the stir-fry vegetables, and cook until just cooked through, with a little crunch to them, 5 minutes. In the final 2 minutes, stir in your chosen protein. Season to taste.

3. Place on top of your whole grains of choice and sprinkle with sesame seeds (if using).

Note This stir-fry works well with tofu and wheat berries or barley.

Storage This keeps in the fridge for up to 3 days.

Thai-Inspired Stir-Fry

Plant Points 8.25

Serves **2** Prep **5 minutes** Cook **2 to 5 minutes**

 FODMAP-Lite   **Fridge Raid**

Cuisine Flavor Base
4 scallions, roughly chopped
1 lemongrass stalk, roughly chopped, or
   1 teaspoon lemongrass paste
10 cilantro sprigs
2 garlic cloves, roughly chopped
1½ tablespoons peeled, roughly chopped
   fresh ginger
3 tablespoons oyster sauce
1 tablespoon fish sauce
1 tablespoon extra virgin olive oil
Sea salt
Fresh ground black pepper

Additional Vegetables (optional)
1½ cups (100 g) sugar snap peas

To Serve (optional)
Juice of 1 lime (about 1½ tablespoons),
   or to taste
Fresh basil or Thai basil, to taste

1. To make the cuisine flavor base, place the scallions, lemongrass, cilantro, garlic, ginger, oyster sauce, and fish sauce in a high-speed blender and blend until smooth, 1 to 2 minutes. Heat the oil in a medium frying pan or wok over medium heat. Add the sauce and cook until warmed through, for 1 minute.

2. Add in the stir-fry vegetables mix (and additional vegetables, if using). Cook until the veggies are just cooked, still with a little crunch to them, 5 minutes. In the final 2 minutes, stir in your protein and whole grains of choice. Season to taste. Top with the lime juice and fresh herbs to taste (if using).

Note This stir-fry works well with butter beans and rice noodles.

Storage This keeps in the fridge for up to 3 days.

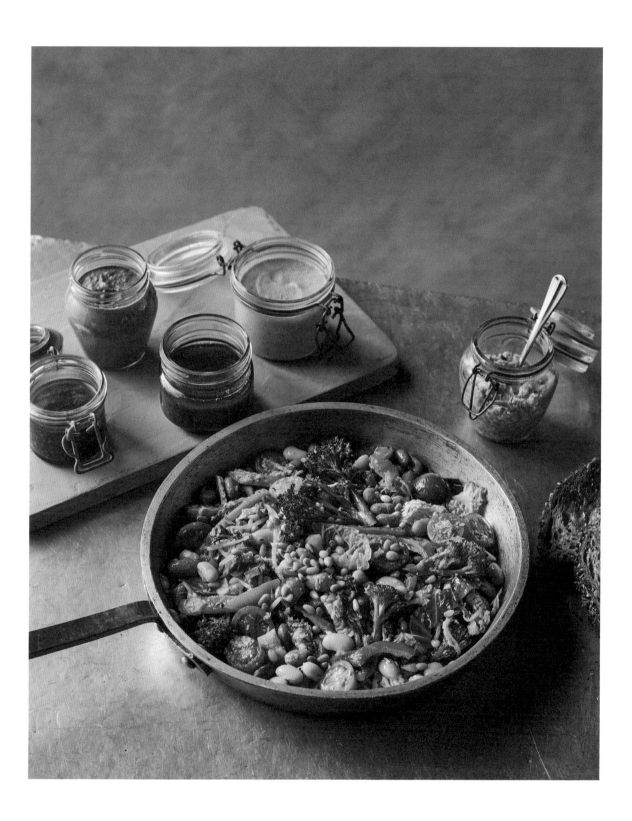

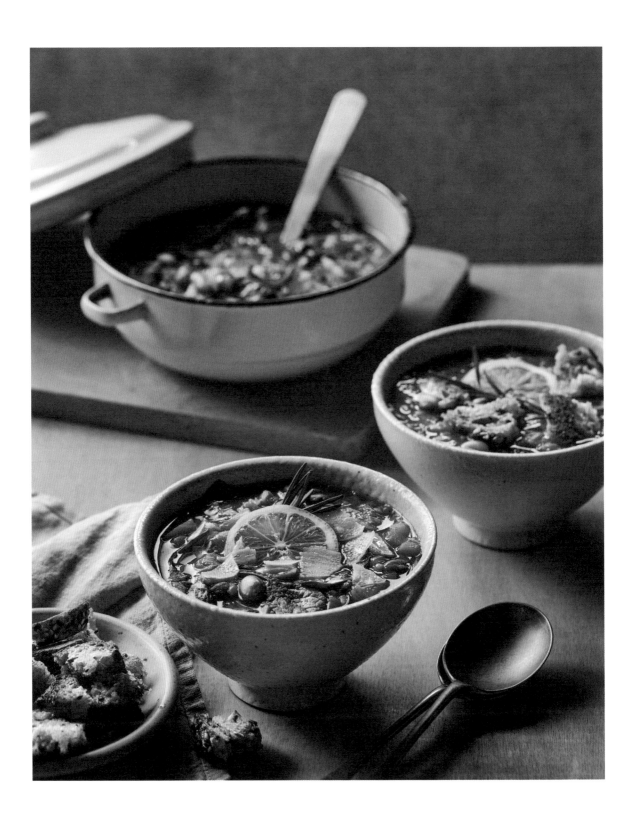

Mediterranean Hug Soup

Plant Points
10.75

Serves **4**   Prep **10 minutes**   Cook **40 minutes**

 Freezer

Everything that's great about the Mediterranean captured in a bowl. The heart-warming atmosphere, the flavors, the comfort . . . and, of course, the good gut health. With nearly half your daily fiber needs and a load of prebiotics, your microbes will fall in love with the Med way of life, too.

Two 15-ounce (425 g) cans mixed beans, drained and rinsed

½ cup (50 g) freekeh or whole grain of choice

1 fresh rosemary sprig or ½ teaspoon of dried rosemary

2 bay leaves

Sea salt

Fresh ground black pepper

1 tablespoon extra virgin olive oil

2 leeks, roughly chopped

2 celery stalks, roughly chopped

1 large carrot, roughly chopped

2 garlic cloves, roughly chopped

One 14.5-ounce (411 g) can diced tomatoes

1½ quarts (1.5 L) vegetable stock

1⅔ cup (50 g) baby spinach leaves, roughly chopped

To Serve (optional)

2 tablespoons extra virgin olive oil

1 slice seeded sourdough bread or bread of choice, torn into pieces

2 fresh rosemary sprigs, halved

Parmesan, grated or shaved

½ lemon, sliced into 4 rounds

1. Heat the olive oil in a large saucepan over medium-high heat and add the leeks, celery, carrots, and garlic, then cook until softened, 5 minutes.

2. Remove from the heat and add the diced tomatoes. Using an immersion blender, blend to form a coarse mixture, about 30 seconds.

3. Add the beans, freekeh, rosemary, and bay leaves. Pour in the vegetable stock. Season to taste, then bring up to a gentle boil.

4. Cover and cook until the freekeh is tender, about 35 minutes. Stir occasionally to prevent sticking and add a splash of water if you prefer a thinner soup.

5. A few minutes before the soup is ready, heat 2 tablespoons of olive oil in a frying pan over medium heat. Add the bread (if using) to the pan and fry until lightly toasted, about 2 minutes.

6. When the soup is ready, remove the bay leaves and add the spinach leaves, stirring to wilt. Season to taste.

7. Ladle into bowls and top each one with the croutons, rosemary, Parmesan, and lemon (if using).

Switch In the summer months, try swapping the rosemary for some fresh basil or parsley as a lighter alternative.

Storage This soup can be refrigerated for 3 days and frozen for up to 1 month.

Tip Short on time? Try quick-cook grains, which are available at most grocery stores.

Phyllo Parcels with Saucy Mushrooms

Plant Points
7.75

Serves **2**   Makes **9 parcels (with about ⅔ cup/160 g left over to make two Reinvented Saucy Mushroom Pita Pockets)**   Prep **15 minutes**   Cook **15 minutes**

The visual appeal of a delicate entrée, with the nourishment and comfort of a main course. These 100 percent plant-based parcels are sure to be a hit with the whole family. And it gets better—page 209 shows you how to turn the leftover mushroom mixture into a tasty lunch the next day.

8 ounces (225 g) mixed mushrooms (e.g., button, portobello, cremini)
1 tablespoon extra virgin olive oil
½ onion, diced
¾ cup (50 g) shredded cabbage or greens of choice
½ cup (50 g) shredded carrot
1 garlic clove, grated or crushed
1 tablespoon harissa
3.5 ounces (100 g) silken tofu, roughly chopped
⅓ cup (75 g) soy yogurt or yogurt of choice
½ cup (50 g) walnuts, chopped
Sea salt
Fresh ground black pepper

Pastry Parcels
4 phyllo sheets
Extra virgin olive oil, for brushing

1. Preheat the oven to 415°F (210°C) and line a baking sheet with parchment paper.

2. Place the mushrooms in a food processor and roughly pulse to form a chunky texture. Heat the oil in a large saucepan over high heat. Add the mushrooms and onions and cook stirring frequently, until the mushrooms have greatly reduced in volume and the liquid has evaporated, 5 minutes.

3. Add the cabbage, carrot, garlic, and harissa, and stir to combine. Cook until the cabbage is just softened, 1 to 2 minutes, then remove from the heat. Add the tofu, yogurt, and walnuts, and stir to combine. Taste and season to preference. Set aside.

4. Unroll the phyllo onto a clean surface and brush two sheets with olive oil. Add another layer of sheets on top of each one, so you have two double sheets. Create an 18 x 18-inch (45 x 45 cm) square, overlapping the two double sheets as needed. Brush the overlapping areas with the oil to help them stick.

5. Cut the square into three columns and three rows, making nine squares. Place a spoonful (about 1.5 ounces/40 g) in the middle of each section of pastry, brush around the filling with a little olive oil, then gently pull up the edges to make a parcel. Scrunch into place.

6. Place them on the baking sheet and bake for 10 minutes or until the phyllo is a deep golden brown.

Storage These are best eaten warm out of the oven so the phyllo stays crispy. They will keep in the fridge for up to 3 days. Reheat in the oven for 5 minutes to get that phyllo crunch back.

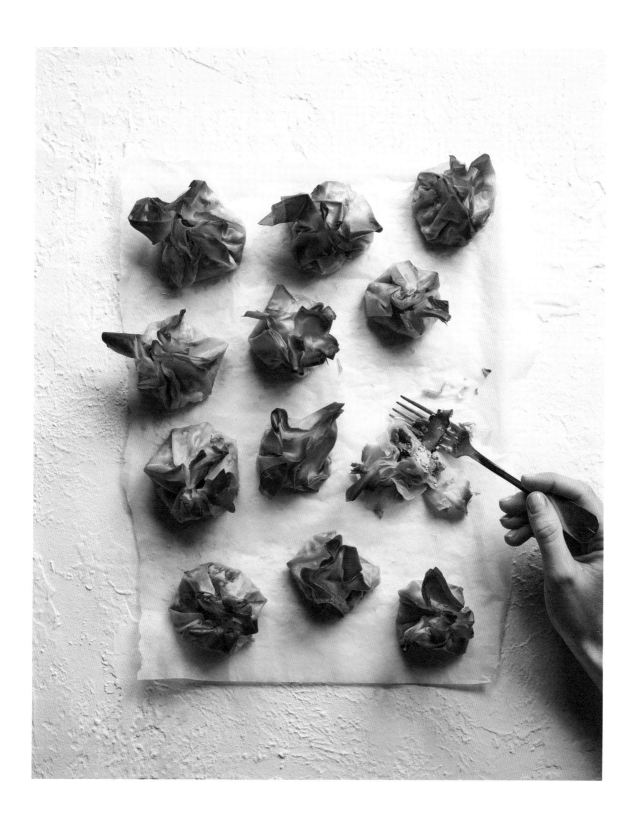

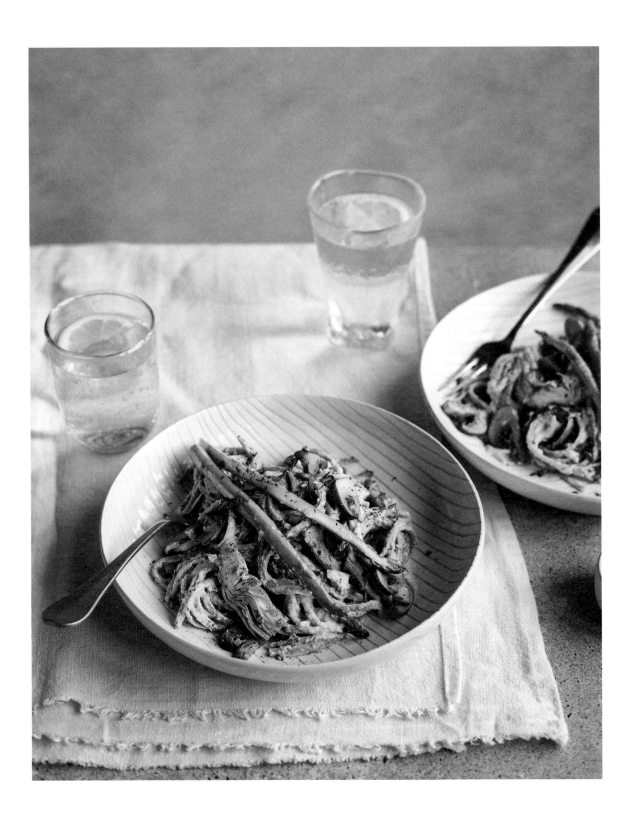

Creamy Dairy-Free Linguine

Plant Points
7.25

Serves **4**   Prep **10 minutes**   Cook **15 minutes**

 Zero Waste

Turns out it *is* possible to make a creamy pasta with nothing but plants. The silken tofu and cashew cream pair perfectly with the prebiotic artichokes, mushrooms, and asparagus.

Sauce
⅔ cup (90 g) cashews
⅓ cup plus 1 tablespoon
   (95 ml) boiling water
8 ounces (225 g) silken tofu
3 tablespoons nutritional
   yeast
1 teaspoon lemon zest
Juice of ½ lemon (about
   1½ tablespoons)
1⅓ cup (20 g) fresh basil,
   finely chopped

Sea salt
8 ounces (225 g) linguine
   or pasta of choice
2 tablespoons oil from the
   artichoke hearts
1 shallot or ¼ red onion,
   finely chopped
8 ounces (225 g) chestnut
   mushrooms or mushrooms
   of choice, roughly chopped
6 ounces (170 g) artichoke
   hearts, preserved in oil
5 ounces (140 g) asparagus
   spears, halved lengthwise
Fresh ground black pepper

1. Soak the cashews in boiling water. Set aside for at least 10 minutes.

2. Bring a large saucepan of water to a boil and add a big pinch of salt. Add the pasta and cook for 10 minutes (or according to package instructions).

3. While the pasta is cooking, heat 2 tablespoons of the oil from the artichoke hearts in a large frying pan over medium-high heat and add the shallot. Cook for 2 minutes, then add the mushrooms, artichoke hearts, and asparagus. Cook over medium-high heat for 5 minutes, or until the mushrooms are golden brown and the asparagus is al dente, about 5 minutes. Set aside a third of this mixture to add on top of the plated dish.

4. Place the cashews and their water, the tofu, nutritional yeast, lemon zest, and lemon juice in a high-powered food processor. Blend until smooth, scraping the sides down occasionally, for about 5 minutes. Stir in the basil and season to taste.

5. Drain the pasta (reserving a couple of spoonfuls of pasta water) and add it to the veggies in the pan along with the sauce. Toss to combine, adding a splash of the reserved pasta water to thin the sauce if needed.

6. Heat through for a minute or so, divide among serving dishes, and finish with a grind of black pepper and any reserved mushroom mixture.

Tip Using the oil from jars of preserved veggies (like the artichoke hearts) can add a real kick of flavor, as the veggies have marinated in and flavored it—plus there's zero waste!

Switch Want an extra plant point? Add ⅓ cup (50 g) pine nuts in the final 2 minutes of the veggies' cooking.

Storage The sauce will keep in the fridge for up to 1 week. The whole dish will keep for up to 3 days in the fridge.

Orange-Glazed Roasted Salmon

Plant Points
13.25

Serves **4**   Prep **10 minutes**   Cook **20 minutes**

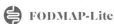 **FODMAP-Lite**

A celebration of omega-3: one nutrient many of us overlook for gut health. This roasted salmon with orange glaze is the perfect reminder that health and flavor absolutely can go hand in hand. If you have the extra time, it's best served with a side of Sticky Parsnips (page 266) along with the whole grains and greens. If you're making the parsnips, triple the marinade.

4 skin-on salmon fillets (4.5 to
    5 ounces/130 to 150 g each)
½ tablespoon soy sauce
1 tablespoon toasted sesame oil
14 ounces (400 g) greens of choice
    (e.g., bok choy, mixed greens, or kale)
18 ounces (510 g) precooked mixed
    whole grains or whole grains of choice
2 scallions, sliced
1 red chile, seeded and finely sliced
    (optional)

Marinade
Juice of ½ orange (about 3 tablespoons)
1½ tablespoon soy sauce
1 Medjool date, mixed to a paste (see
    page 136) or 1 tablespoon sweetener
    of choice
1½ teaspoons sesame oil
1 garlic clove, grated
2 teaspoons peeled, grated ginger

To Serve
Sticky Parsnips (page 266, optional)
1 tablespoon sesame seeds

1. Preheat the oven to 425°F (220°C).

2. To make the marinade, place the orange juice, soy sauce, date paste, sesame oil, garlic, and ginger in a small saucepan and bring to a boil, stirring frequently, until reduced and syrupy, about 5 minutes.

3. Meanwhile, make four little foil "bowls" for the salmon to go in and place them on a baking sheet. Add one piece of salmon to each "bowl" and coat with the reduced marinade, then fold up the foil.

4. Bake for 10 minutes, opening the foil for the final 5 minutes to allow the salmon to brown a little. The salmon is done when the flesh is opaque all the way through; if it still looks translucent, return to the oven for 2 more minutes.

5. While the fish is in the oven, heat the soy sauce and sesame oil in a frying pan over medium heat before adding the greens. Cook until softened, about 5 minutes.

6. Add the whole grains, scallions, and chile (if using) to the pan and heat through for few minutes.

7. Divide the whole grains among serving plates, along with the Sticky Parsnips (if using), and top with the greens, salmon, and any juices from the foil bowls. Sprinkle with sesame seeds.

Tip Want crispy salmon skin? Finish the salmon off in the frying pan over medium heat, skin-side down, for the last 5 minutes.

Storage This will keep in the fridge for up to 3 days.

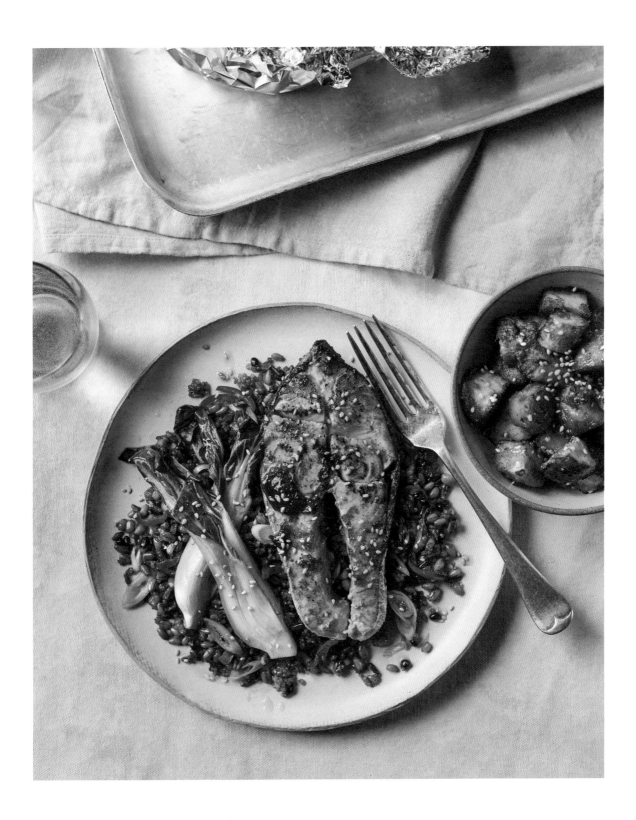

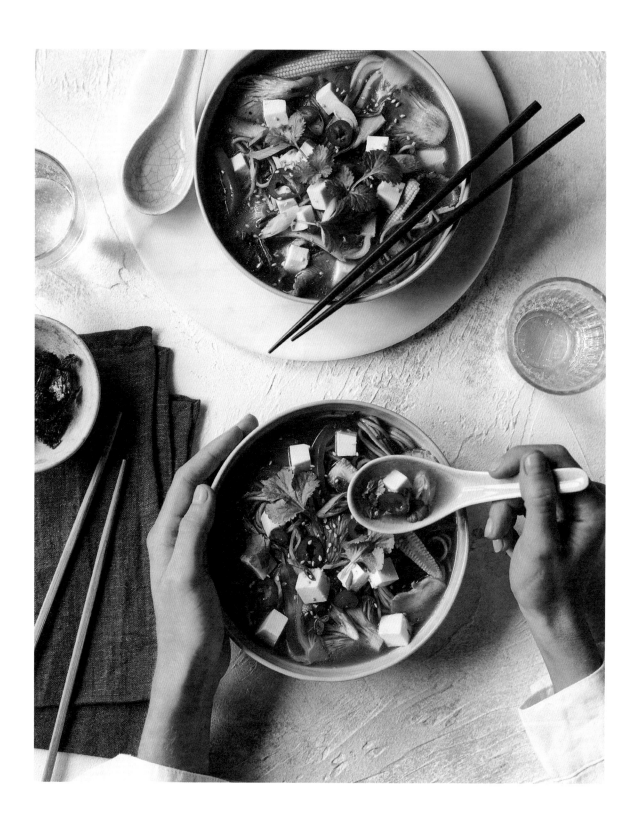

Easy Noodle Soup

Serves **2**   Prep **10 minutes**   Cook **10 minutes**

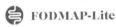 **FODMAP-Lite**

Craving a pot of noodles? Let me tempt you with this flavorful soup that will leave you and your microbes feeling warm and fuzzy inside. It's also a great way to use up any leftover veggies, as the broth will give them a new lease of life.

1 quart (1 L) vegetable stock
½ ounce (15 g) ginger
1 tablespoon soy sauce
2 whole star anise
10 cilantro sprigs
5 ounces (150 g) dried soba noodles,
    10 ounces (300 g) cooked soba
    noodles, or noodles of choice
5 ounces (150 g) bok choy, halved
    lengthwise
1 tablespoon sesame oil
5 ounces (150 g) oyster mushrooms
6 baby corn, halved lengthwise
½ red bell pepper, sliced
8 ounces (225 g) silken tofu, cut into
    bite-size cubes

To Serve
1 red chile, thinly sliced, to taste
1 scallion, thinly sliced
1½ teaspoons sesame seeds
½ teaspoon nori flakes (optional)

1. Heat the stock in a large saucepan over medium heat. Add the ginger, soy sauce, and star anise.

2. Finely chop the cilantro stems and add them to the stock, saving the leaves for garnish. Bring the stock to a boil, simmer for 5 minutes, then add the noodles and cook according to package instructions (about 5 minutes). Add the bok choy for the final 2 minutes.

3. While the noodles are cooking, heat the sesame oil in a frying pan and, when hot, add the mushrooms, corn, and bell pepper. Cook until softened, stirring frequently, for 5 minutes.

4. Divide the noodles and bok choy between two bowls and pour the broth over the top (discard the ginger and star anise). Add the tofu (it will warm through in the broth) and divide the vegetable mixture between the two bowls.

5. Sprinkle with the chile, scallion, sesame seeds, and nori flakes (if using), and add the reserved cilantro leaves on top.

Storage   This is best eaten immediately but can be kept in the fridge for 2 days.

Green Pea and "Ham" Soup

Plant Points
11.25

Serves **4**   Prep **10 minutes**   Cook **10 minutes**

 Freezer

A plant-based play on ham and pea soup. This color-popping creamy soup delivers around half your daily fiber needs per portion. The crispy coconut "ham," hint of mint, and sweetness from the peas takes things to the next level. And the appeal doesn't stop there—it's also perfect for warming your hands around on a winter's day.

1 tablespoon extra virgin olive oil
1 onion, chopped
3 celery stalks, chopped
3 garlic cloves, sliced
One 15-ounce (425 g) can white
   beans, drained
2⅔ cups (400 g) frozen peas
5 cups (150 g) baby spinach leaves
⅓ cup (5 g) mint leaves, or more
   to taste
3½ cups (840 ml) vegetable stock, hot
Sea salt
Fresh ground black pepper

Coconut "Ham"
½ cup (30 g) coconut flakes
1 teaspoon extra virgin olive oil
½ teaspoon smoked paprika
¼ teaspoon garlic powder

To Serve (optional)
Generous ⅓ cup (100 g)
   probiotic yogurt
4 slices Foolproof Fermented Wheaten
   Bread (page 178) or crusty bread
   of choice

1. Preheat the oven to 400°F (200°C) and line a baking sheet with parchment paper.

2. Heat the olive oil in a large saucepan over medium-low heat and add the onion, celery, and garlic. Cook until softened but not browned, about 5 minutes.

3. While the veggies are cooking, place the coconut flakes, 1 teaspoon of olive oil, paprika, garlic powder, and a pinch of salt onto the baking sheet and toss until the coconut is coated. Bake for 3 to 4 minutes, until the coconut is golden brown.

4. Once the onion and celery have softened, add the beans, peas, spinach, mint, and stock, and stir to combine. Bring to a boil, then simmer for a few minutes.

5. Remove from the heat and blend with an immersion blender to your preferred consistency. Season to taste.

6. Divide the soup among the bowls and top with the yogurt (if using), swirl it with a knife, and add some of the coconut "ham." Serve with bread.

Storage This soup can be kept in the fridge for up to 3 days, or frozen for up to 1 month.

Tip For extra-smooth soup, blend in a high-powered blender for 1 to 2 minutes before adding the yogurt and serving.

Loaded Vegan Nachos

Serves **4**   Prep **10–20 minutes** + Soak **30 minutes (optional)**

Cook **15 minutes**

There are few things more satisfying than a tray of loaded nachos with all the trimmings. This is one of my favorites for a fun Friday night. The cashew cheese, guacamole, and meaty jackfruit combo makes it hard to stop—but you are eating for trillions of microbes, after all.

4 whole wheat pitas (about 6 inches/15 cm)
2 tablespoons extra virgin olive oil
Sea salt

Pulled Jackfruit
2 tablespoons extra virgin olive oil
1 tablespoon honey
1 tablespoon soy sauce
1 teaspoon ground cumin
1 teaspoon garlic powder
1 teaspoon smoked paprika
½ teaspoon Worcestershire sauce
¼ teaspoon fresh ground black pepper
Pinch of cayenne (optional)
One 14-ounce (397 g) can jackfruit, drained
One 14.5-ounce (425 g) can black beans, drained and rinsed
Sea salt
Fresh ground black pepper

Guacamole
1 avocado
Juice from 1 lime (about 1½ tablespoons)
3 tablespoons chopped cilantro
1 teaspoon extra virgin olive oil (optional)
Sea salt
Fresh ground black pepper

Cashew Cheese (optional)
1 cup plus 3 tablespoons (155 g) cashews, soaked in 1¼ cups (300 ml) boiling water for at least 30 minutes
3 tablespoons nutritional yeast
2 teaspoons lemon juice
1 teaspoon Dijon mustard
½ teaspoon garlic powder
¼ teaspoon smoked paprika
¼ teaspoon ground turmeric

To Serve (optional):
¼ cup (60 ml) Garlicky Aquafaba Aioli (page 172) or yogurt
1 jalapeño, sliced
½ bunch cilantro, roughly chopped
⅔ cup (100 g) cherry tomatoes, halved
2 limes, cut into wedges

1. Preheat the oven to 400°F (200°C), and line a baking sheet with parchment paper.

2. Cut the pitas in half so you have two ovals, and then cut into "tortilla chips." Drizzle with the olive oil and season with salt. Place on the baking sheet and bake for 10 minutes or until crisp.

3. While the chips are baking, make the pulled jackfruit. In a medium bowl, mix together the olive oil, honey, soy sauce, cumin, garlic powder, paprika, Worcestershire sauce, black pepper, and cayenne. Shred the jackfruit with your hands, then add to the bowl and coat with the mixture. Set aside to marinate.

4. To make the guacamole, cut the avocado in half and remove the pit. Spoon the flesh into a small bowl and press with a fork until coarsely mashed. Mix in the cilantro, lime juice, and olive oil (if using) and season to taste. Set aside.

5. To make the cashew cheese (if using), place the cashews and their soaking water, nutritional yeast, lemon juice, mustard, garlic powder, paprika, and turmeric in a high-powered blender. Blend until smooth, scraping the sides down occasionally, 3 to 4 minutes.

6. Heat a frying pan over medium heat, add the marinated jackfruit, and cook until slightly charred, 3 to 5 minutes, adding a splash of water if the jackfruit becomes too dry. Add the black beans for the last minute, then remove from the heat.

7. Take the baking sheet out of the oven and top the warm pita chips with the jackfruit, cashew cheese, and guacamole, along with whatever toppings you'd like: aioli, jalapeño slices, cilantro, tomatoes, and/or limes. Serve any remaining cheese in a bowl on the side.

Storage   The pulled jackfruit will keep in the fridge for up to 3 days, and the cashew cheese will keep well in a sealed container in the fridge for up to 5 days, but the loaded nachos are best eaten immediately.

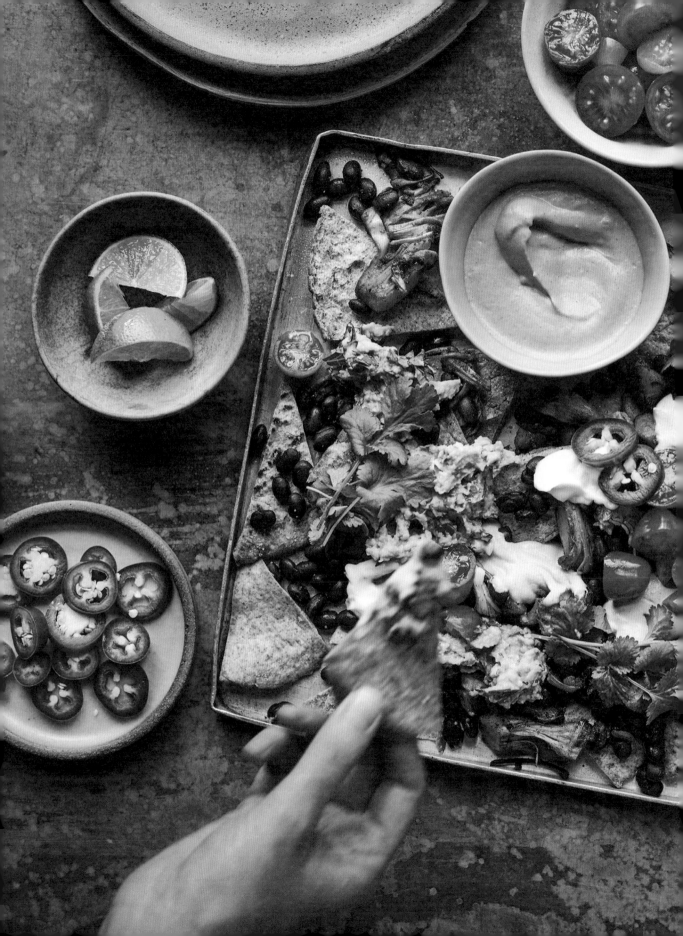

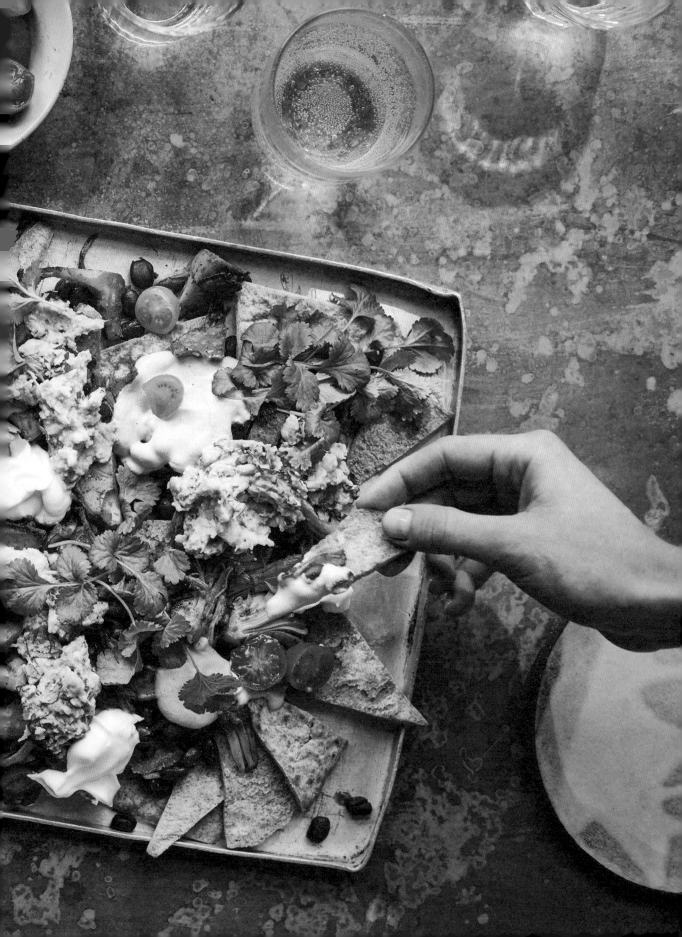

Fancy Dinners

Hearty Lasagna
239

Spicy Red Lentil Bowl
242

Creamy Beans with "Meaty" Jackfruit
245

Sweet Potato Gnocchi with Sprout Pesto
246

Spinach and Ricotta Stuffed Shells
249

Tear-and-Share Bread with Butter Bean Relish
250

Rainbow Roast with Green Yorkshire Puddings
253

Barley Butternut Risotto
254

Bangers and Mash, Revamped
257

Chicken 'n' Veggie Meatballs
258

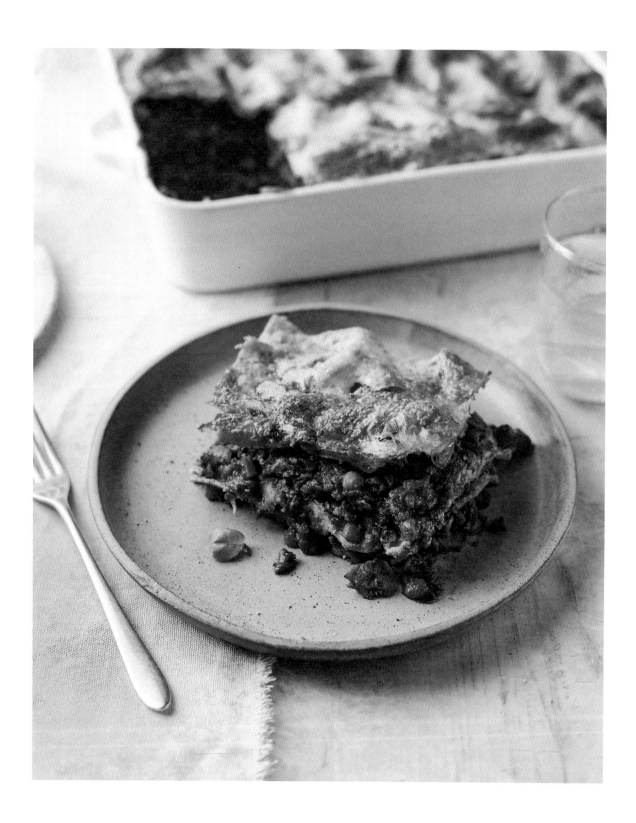

Hearty Lasagna

Plant Points
9.25

Serves **8**   Prep **20 minutes**   Cook **1 hour**

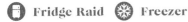 **Fridge Raid** **Freezer**

This is the ideal dish to show meat lovers that eating more plants doesn't mean missing out. A comforting family staple that ticks all the flavor boxes with half (or none) of the meat. The versatile ragu can be frozen and used as the base for shepherd's pie or simply poured over pasta—this is so much more than your average lasagna!

Ragù

2 tablespoons extra virgin olive oil
2 carrots, diced
2 celery stalks, diced
1 onion, chopped
4 garlic cloves, grated or minced
14 ounces (400 g) chestnut mushrooms or mushrooms of choice
8 ounces (225 g) ground beef (optional)
2 tablespoons tomato paste
One 15-ounce (425 g) can green lentils, drained and rinsed (or two if not using beef)
Two 14.5-ounce (411 g) cans diced tomatoes
⅔ cup (10 g) fresh basil, finely chopped
1 tablespoon balsamic vinegar
1 tablespoon Italian seasoning
½ teaspoon ground nutmeg
Sea salt
Fresh ground black pepper

White Sauce

2 tablespoons extra virgin olive oil
⅓ cup (45 g) all-purpose flour or flour of choice
3 cups (720 ml) soy milk or milk of choice
⅓ cup (30 g) grated Parmesan or cheese of choice
1 teaspoon Dijon mustard
Sea salt
Fresh ground black pepper

To Assemble

Olive oil, for greasing
1 pound (450 g) dried whole wheat lasagna noodles or lasagna noodles of choice
1⅓ cups (40 g) baby spinach leaves
⅓ cup (40 g) grated cheddar or cheese of choice
⅓ cup (5 g) fresh basil

1. To make the ragù, heat the olive oil in a large saucepan over medium heat. Add the carrots, celery, onion, and garlic, and cook until softened and starting to brown.

2. While the veggies are cooking, pulse the mushrooms in a food processor until finely chopped, then set aside.

3. Add the meat (if using) to the pan, then add the tomato paste and cook until the meat is browned, about 5 minutes. If omitting the meat, add the tomato paste along with the mushrooms, tomatoes, lentils, basil, vinegar, Italian seasoning, and nutmeg.

4. Stir well, then bring to a boil. Reduce the heat, cover, and gently simmer until reduced slightly, 15 minutes. Stir occasionally to prevent the sauce from sticking on the bottom of the pan. Season to taste.

5. While the ragù is cooking, make the white sauce. Heat the olive oil in a saucepan over medium-low heat. Add the flour and stir continuously to form a roux, 2 minutes. Slowly whisk in the milk. Bring to a boil, then reduce to a simmer until thickened, 5 minutes. Remove from the heat, whisk in the Parmesan and mustard, and season to taste.

6. When you're ready to assemble the lasagna, preheat the oven to 350°F (180°C) and lightly oil an 11 x 7-inch (28 x 18 cm) baking dish. ➡

7. Spread one third of the ragù over the bottom of the dish, then add a layer of lasagna noodles (breaking them to fit, if needed), followed by a layer of white sauce. Top with half of the spinach. Repeat these layers two more times, but instead of a third layer of spinach leaves, sprinkle the cheddar over the final layer of white sauce.

8. Cover with foil and bake for 30 minutes, removing the foil in the final 10 minutes to crisp up the top. Garnish with basil leaves before serving.

Eggplant Lasagna

Already had pasta this week? Try switching the lasagna noodles for eggplant layers.

3 medium eggplants (about 26 ounces/750 g)
2 tablespoons extra virgin olive oil
Sea salt
Fresh ground black pepper

1. To prepare the eggplant layers, preheat the oven to 425°F (220°C) and line two large baking sheets with parchment paper.

2. While the ragù is cooking, thinly slice the eggplant into ⅛-inch (3 mm) thick slices (using a mandolin if possible). Lay as many as you can in a single layer on the baking sheets. Brush lightly with olive oil, season, and bake for 8 to 10 minutes, until softened and browning in patches. Repeat with the remaining slices.

3. Cook the ragù until thickened, about 10 more minutes, as the eggplant doesn't absorb as much liquid as the noodles. Layer the lasagna as described in Hearty Lasagna (page 239), using the eggplant slices in place of the noodles.

Note You can serve the ragù by itself over pasta, or use it in a cottage pie—just add 2 tablespoons of Worcestershire sauce instead of the balsamic vinegar and leave out the fresh basil.

Storage This lasagna will keep for 3 days in the fridge or 2 months in the freezer uncooked; defrost fully in the fridge overnight and bake according to recipe directions.

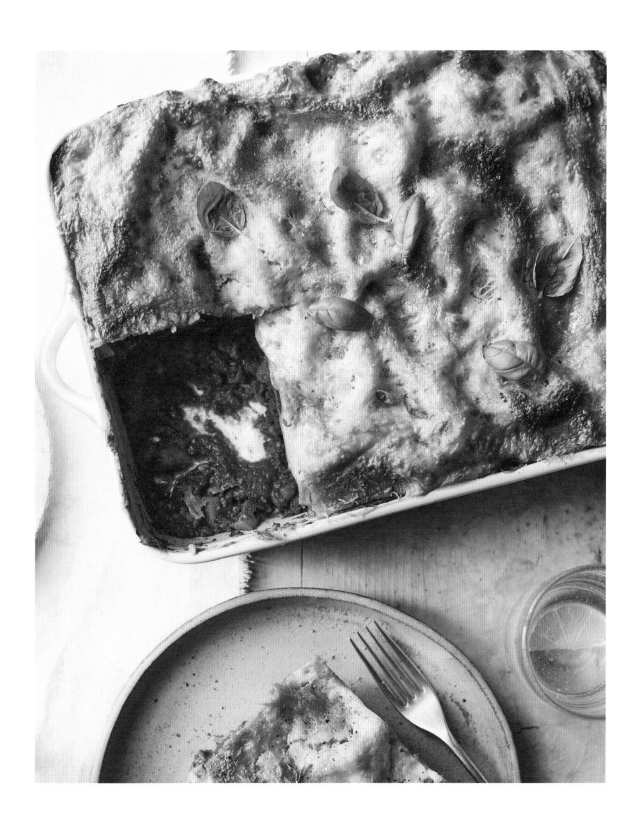

Spicy Red Lentil Bowl

Plant Points
10

Serves **4**   Prep **15 minutes**   Cook **25 minutes**

 Freezer

This recipe was inspired by my love of dal and has evolved over the years into this delicious dish with added texture and flavor from the roasted toppings. Serving up to 40 percent of your daily fiber needs, this is one tasty way to thriving gut microbes.

2 tablespoons extra virgin olive oil
1 green chile, chopped
3 garlic cloves, grated
2 teaspoons peeled, grated fresh ginger
8 curry leaves
1 teaspoon ground cumin
1 teaspoon ground turmeric
1⅔ cups (250 g) split red lentils
2 cups (140 g) shredded cabbage
One 14.5-ounce (411 g) can
    diced tomatoes
1⅔ cups (400 ml) coconut milk
1⅔ cups (400 ml) vegetable stock
1⅓ cup (40 g) spinach, roughly
    chopped (optional)
Sea salt
Fresh ground black pepper

Roasted Vegetables
2 sweet potatoes
One 14.5-ounce (425 g) can chickpeas,
    drained and rinsed
2 red onions, cut into 8 wedges
2 tablespoons extra virgin olive oil
2 teaspoons curry powder
Sea salt
Fresh ground black pepper

To Serve
¼ cup (60 g) probiotic yogurt
½ cup (30 g) coconut flakes, toasted
1 small bunch cilantro, roughly chopped

1. Preheat the oven to 425°F (220°C). Line a baking sheet with parchment paper.

2. Place the sweet potatoes in a microwave-safe dish with a splash of water and cook on high for 5 minutes to soften.

3. Meanwhile, heat 2 tablespoons of oil in a large saucepan over medium heat and add the chile, garlic, ginger, curry leaves, cumin, and turmeric. Cook until aromatic, 2 to 3 minutes. If the spices stick, add 1 to 2 tablespoons of water.

4. Add the lentils and cabbage and stir well to coat them in the spices, then mix in the tomatoes, coconut milk, and stock. Bring to a gentle boil.

5. Reduce the heat, cover, and cook until the lentils are tender, about 20 minutes. In the final minute, stir in the spinach (if using). Taste and adjust seasoning to preference. Add extra vegetable stock if it's too thick.

6. While the lentils are cooking, transfer the softened sweet potatoes, along with the chickpeas and onions, to a baking sheet and drizzle with 2 tablespoons of olive oil. Sprinkle with curry powder and season to taste. Toss to combine, then bake for 20 minutes or until golden brown.

7. Serve topped with the roasted veggies and the yogurt, coconut flakes, and cilantro (if using).

Tip It's easy to toast your own coconut flakes! All it takes is 1 to 2 minutes in a frying pan over medium heat. Be sure to stir the flakes every few seconds to ensure even toasting.

Switch Had enough sweet potato this week? Switch it out for eggplant or zucchini (no need to microwave the zucchini).

Storage This will keep in the fridge for up to 3 days or in the freezer for 1 month.

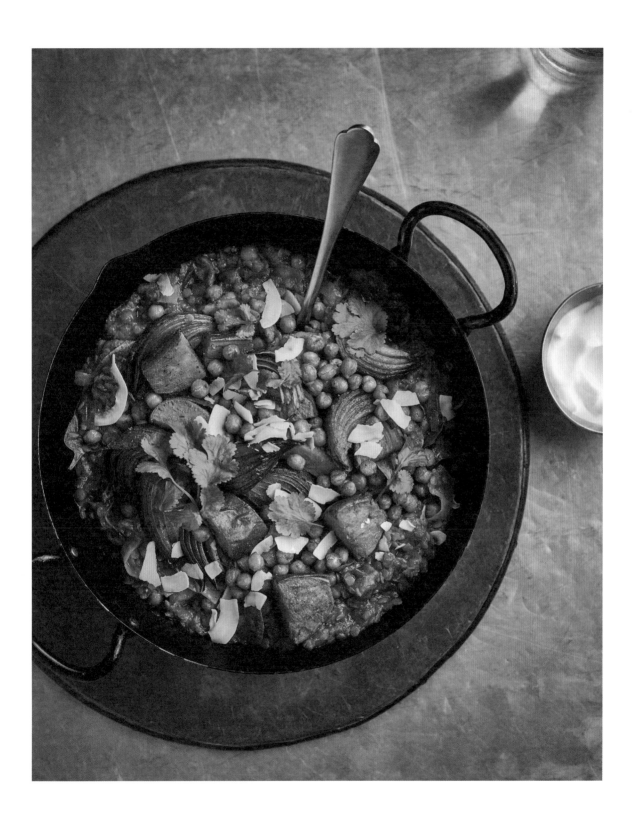

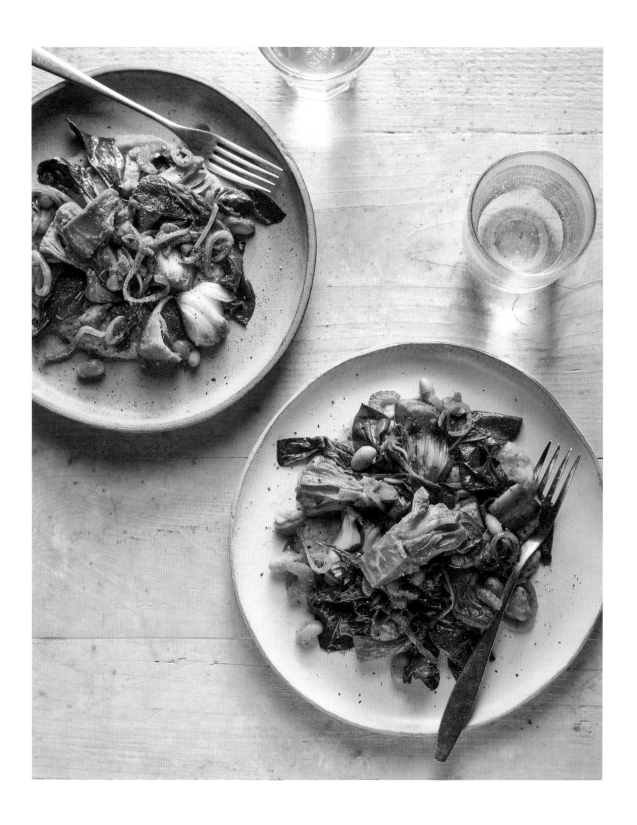

Creamy Beans with "Meaty" Jackfruit

Plant Points 5.75

Serves **2**   Prep **10 minutes**   Cook **15 minutes**

Forget those processed mock meats and say hello to naturally "meaty" jackfruit. This hearty (and gut-loving) dish has a prebiotic punch from the bean base and is better than your average bean stew.

Marinade

2 tablespoons extra virgin olive oil
1 tablespoon Worcestershire sauce
1 teaspoon Marmite or miso paste
½ teaspoon dried rosemary
¼ teaspoon onion powder

One 20-ounce (565 g) can jackfruit,
  drained, rinsed and patted dry
  (drained weight 10 ounces/280 g)
1 tablespoon extra virgin olive oil
1 small white onion, sliced
2 celery stalks, sliced
2 garlic cloves, grated
1 cup (240 ml) vegetable stock
One 15-ounce (425 g) can cannellini
  beans, drained and rinsed
0.75 ounce (20 g) Parmesan, grated
2 cups (60 g) spinach or mixed greens
Sea salt
Fresh ground black pepper

1. To make the marinade, combine the olive oil, Worcestershire sauce, marmite, rosemary, and onion powder in a medium bowl. Add the jackfruit and stir to coat. Leave to marinate for a few minutes.

2. Heat 1 tablespoon olive oil in a frying pan over medium heat. Add the onion, celery, and garlic, and cook until softened and golden brown, 5 minutes.

3. Transfer half of the vegetable mixture to a high-powered blender, along with the vegetable stock and half of the beans, then blend until smooth. Set aside the other half of the vegetable mixture.

4. Return the blended mixture to the frying pan, along with the Parmesan, and simmer until the stock has reduced significantly, 10 to 15 minutes. Season to taste.

5. While the vegetable mixture is simmering, heat a small frying pan over medium heat. Add the jackfruit with its marinade. Cook, stirring frequently, until the marinade has reduced and the jackfruit is browned, 5 to 10 minutes. In the final few minutes, add the reserved (non-pureed) vegetable mixture and beans. Stir-fry until thoroughly combined, a few minutes, then add the greens. When the greens have wilted (1 to 2 minutes), you're ready to serve.

6. Divide the pureed vegetable mixture between bowls, then top with the jackfruit stir-fry mixture and finish with grind of black pepper.

Switch No jackfruit? Switch it out for 11 ounces (310 g) of mushrooms.

Storage This will keep for 3 days in the fridge.

Sweet Potato Gnocchi with Sprout Pesto

Plant Points
6.75

Serves **4 to 6**   Prep **30 minutes**   Cook **20 minutes**

❄ **Freezer**

Feeling a little adventurous, but not ready to make pasta from scratch? Foolproof for the novice cook, gnocchi are great for building your pasta-making confidence. Pan-frying makes them deliciously crispy, but you can enjoy them straight from the boiling water with the pesto, too.

Gnocchi

4 to 5 medium sweet potatoes (about 23 ounces/650 g)

1 large russet potato (about 12 ounces/ 350 g)

1¼ cup (150 g) spelt flour, plus extra to dust

1 teaspoon ground turmeric

1 large egg, beaten

1⅓ cup (200 g) cherry tomatoes

1 tablespoon extra virgin olive oil, plus extra for frying

Pesto

2 ounces (55 g) Brussels sprouts

½ cup (50 g) walnuts

2⅔ cups (40 g) fresh basil

2 tablespoons fresh lemon juice, or to taste

½ cup (120 ml) extra virgin olive oil

2 ounces (55 g) Parmesan, finely grated

Sea salt

Fresh ground black pepper

To Serve (optional)

Shaved Parmesan

1. Pierce the sweet and russet potatoes with a fork and cook in the microwave on high for 8 to 10 minutes, until cooked through and soft. Let cool.

2. While the potatoes are cooking, make the pesto. Cook the Brussels sprouts in simmering water or until just tender, 3 minutes. Drain and run under cold water to cool.

3. Place the Brussels sprouts, walnuts, and basil in a food processor, and blend to form a rough paste. Continue to pulse while slowly adding the lemon juice, followed by 1 tablespoon oil and then the Parmesan until you're happy with the consistency and flavor. Season to taste.

4. Scrape out the insides of the cooked potatoes into a large bowl and mash them or use a potato ricer. Add the flour, turmeric, and egg and gently mix together with a butter knife, using a cutting action. This will help prevent the dough from getting tough.

5. Divide the dough into quarters and roll each section into ½ inch (1.5 cm) thick ropes on a lightly floured surface. If the dough is too wet to roll, add a little extra flour. Cut into bite-size gnocchi.

6. Bring a large saucepan of salted water to a boil and carefully drop in one third of the gnocchi. Cook until they float to the surface, about 2 minutes. Repeat with the remaining gnocchi.

7. Heat the remaining 1 tablespoon olive oil in a large frying pan over medium heat and add the cooked gnocchi along with the cherry tomatoes. Toss to coat the gnocchi and cook for a few minutes, until they start to brown slightly.

8. Serve topped with shaved Parmesan (if using) and a twist of black pepper.

Storage Leftover pesto can be kept in the fridge for up to 1 week, covered with olive oil or plastic wrap or frozen for up to 3 months. Fresh gnocchi can be kept in the fridge for up to 2 days or frozen for 1 month.

Switch Stir pesto into wild rice, whole wheat pasta, or store-bought gnocchi.

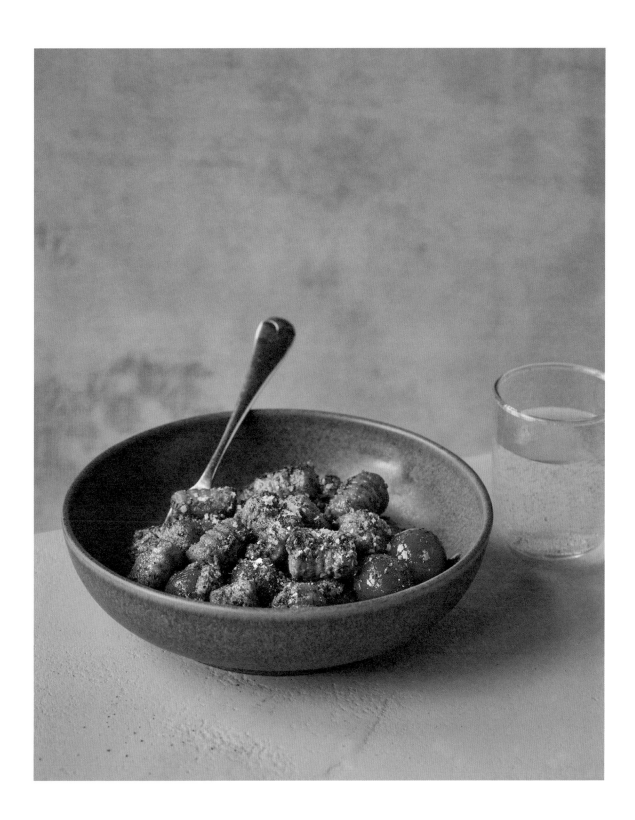

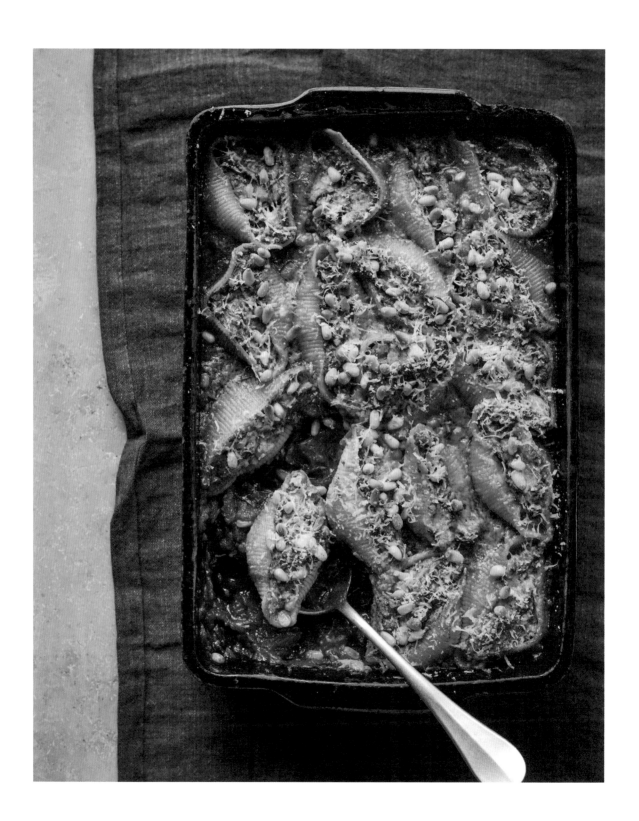

Spinach and Ricotta Stuffed Shells

Plant Points
7.75

Serves **4**   Prep **15 minutes**   Cook **30 minutes**

 FODMAP-Lite   **Freezer**

In my Italian family, homemade ravioli has always been part of our celebrations. But after I moved to London and realized that I didn't have the time or skill to make them myself, I had to choose between forgoing one of my favorites or conjuring up an easier and quicker alternative . . . and so these delicious stuffed shells were born. I couldn't let my microbes miss the feast, so I've ensured that this recipe contains over a third of your daily fiber needs and prebiotics, too.

Tomato Sauce

1 tablespoon extra virgin olive oil
2 garlic cloves, grated
One 14.5-ounce (411 g) can
   diced tomatoes
¾ cup (185 g) tomato puree
10 sun-dried tomato halves, preserved
   in oil, chopped
1⅓ cups (20 g) fresh basil,
   roughly chopped
Sea salt
Fresh ground black pepper

Stuffed Shells

8⅓ cups (250 g) fresh spinach
One 15-ounce (425 g) can mixed beans,
   drained and rinsed
Heaping ¾ cup (115 g) peas,
   fresh or frozen
1 cup (250 g) ricotta
5 ounces (150 g) feta, crumbled
Oil, for greasing
6 ounces (175 g) jumbo shells
2 tablespoons pine nuts
0.75 ounce (20 g) Parmesan, grated

1. To make the tomato sauce, heat the olive oil in a medium saucepan over medium heat and add the garlic. Cook for a couple of minutes until aromatic and then add the diced tomatoes, tomato puree, sun-dried tomatoes, basil, and ½ cup (120 ml) water. Season to taste. Reduce the heat to low and cook until thickened, about 15 minutes.

2. While the sauce cooks, make the pasta filling. Heat a large saucepan over medium heat and add the spinach along with a splash of water. Cover and let the spinach wilt for 2 minutes. Transfer to a sieve and squeeze out the excess water, then place in a food processor. Add the beans and peas, and blend to form a rough mixture, about 2 minutes. Stir in the ricotta and feta.

3. Preheat the oven to 400°F (200°C).

4. Lightly oil a 9 x 13-inch (23 x 33 cm) baking dish. Pour in the tomato sauce and spread out in an even layer.

5. Rinse the saucepan and fill with water. Bring to a boil, then cook the shells for 2 minutes less than the package instructions, so they're just cooked and holding their shape. Drain and, let cool, then stuff with the filling and place all the filled shells in the tomato sauce.

6. Scatter the pine nuts and grated Parmesan over the top and bake for about 20 minutes, until golden brown.

Tip Short on time? Scrap the tomato sauce recipe and use your favorite ready-made tomato-basil pasta sauce.

Storage The cooked shells will keep in the fridge for 3 days. The uncooked filling can keep in the freezer for up to 1 month. Defrost overnight in the fridge, then stuff your shells and cook following the recipe.

Tear-and-Share Bread with Butter Bean Relish

Serves **4**   Prep **10 minutes**   Cook **20 minutes**

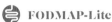 **FODMAP-Lite**

A favorite dinner party dish that everyone can dig into. This crispy sea-salted bread, encasing a sticky, plant-filled relish and served straight out of the oven, will be the talk of the table. It's the perfect opening to introduce your guests to their inner universe of microbes, if they're still outsiders.

2 tablespoons extra virgin olive oil, plus extra for drizzling and brushing

1 large onion, finely chopped

1 rosemary sprig, leaves picked and finely chopped

2 Medjool dates, made into a paste (see page 136), or 2 tablespoons sweetener

1 tablespoon balsamic vinegar

1½ teaspoons Worcestershire sauce

Sea salt

One 15-ounce (425 g) can butter beans, drained and rinsed

One 14.5-ounce (411 g) can diced tomatoes

0.75 ounce (20 g) Parmesan (optional), plus extra for topping

1 teaspoon whole grain mustard

½ teaspoon smoked paprika

1 round bread loaf (about 14 ounces/400 g)

Fresh ground black pepper

1. Preheat the oven to 400°F (200°C).

2. Heat 2 tablespoons olive oil in a medium frying pan over medium-low heat. Add the onion, rosemary, date paste, balsamic vinegar, Worcestershire sauce, and a pinch of salt, and cook until the onions soften and start to brown, about 5 minutes.

3. Add the beans, tomatoes, mustard, and paprika. Cover and bring to a gentle boil until the tomatoes have broken down, 15 minutes. Add up to ½ cup (120 ml) water to thin the mixture if needed. Stir in the Parmesan, if using, in the final minute of cooking.

4. Meanwhile, cut the top off the bread loaf and pull out the insides. Break the top and insides of the loaf into bite-size pieces (these will be used to scoop into the bean mixture). Drizzle the pieces with olive oil, season with salt and pepper, and spread out on a baking sheet. Brush the outside of the loaf with some more olive oil and place it on a second baking sheet. Place both sheets in the oven for 10 minutes or until golden brown.

5. To serve, spoon the bean mixture into the hollowed-out loaf, and serve with the crunchy bread pieces and extra Parmesan (if using).

Storage   The beans will keep in the fridge for up to 3 days and up to 1 month in the freezer.

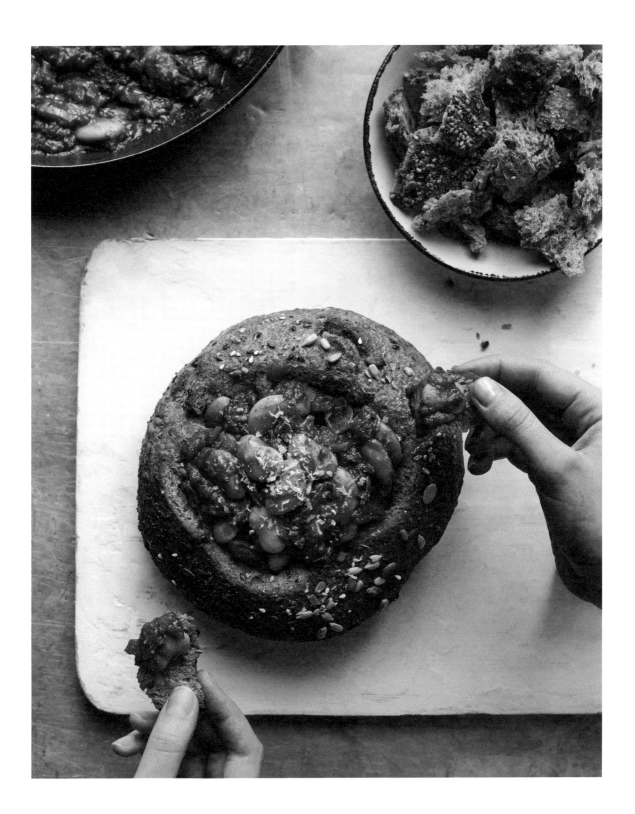

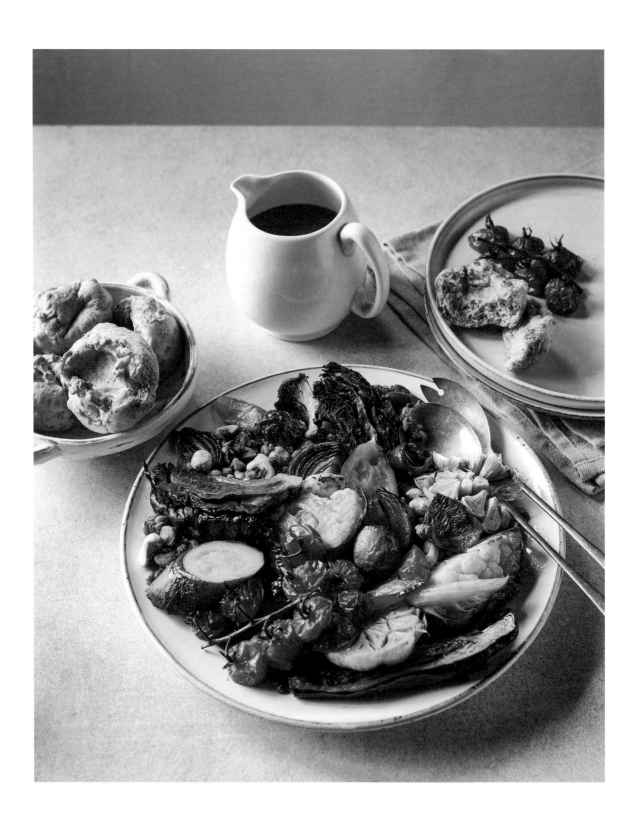

Rainbow Roast with Green Yorkshire Puddings

Plant Points
21.5

Serves **4 (with leftover veggies to make my Reinvented Couscous Salad, page 210)**

Prep **20 minutes**   Cook **55 minutes**

 Fridge Raid   **Freezer**

This is my veggie-forward take on the traditional British Sunday roast. Complete with Yorkshire pudding and gravy, this dish is not only gut-warming but also gives you a head start with your weekly plant points. I make a double batch most Sundays so that a supply of roasted vegetables is ready for the week ahead. Use whatever veggies you've got on hand—I've listed my favorites below.

Roasted Vegetables
1 eggplant, quartered
½ cauliflower, quartered
1 large zucchini, quartered
½ small cabbage, quartered
1 bell pepper, quartered
2 carrots, halved
1 red onion, quartered
10 small tomatoes, ideally on the vine
4 oyster mushrooms or mushrooms of choice
1 whole head of garlic, unpeeled and halved widthwise
2 tablespoons extra virgin olive oil
Sea salt
Fresh ground black pepper

Toppings (optional)
9 ounces (255 g) precooked mixed whole grains
¾ cup (75 g) mixed nuts, or nut of choice
2 tablespoons mixed seeds

Green Yorkshire Puddings
1 tablespoon plus 1 teaspoon sunflower oil
½ cup (70 g) all-purpose flour
½ cup (120 ml) soy milk or milk of choice
2 large eggs
½ cup (15 g) baby spinach
1 tablespoon poppy seeds

To Serve
1 cup (240 ml) Wild Mushroom Gravy (page 272) or gravy of choice

1. Preheat the oven to 400°F (200°C). Line two baking sheets with parchment paper. Spread the eggplant, cauliflower, zucchini, cabbage, bell pepper, carrots, onion, mushrooms, and garlic across the baking sheets, drizzle with the olive oil and season with salt and pepper. Place one baking sheet on the oven's middle rack and the other on the bottom rack. Bake for about 50 minutes, turning the veggies after 20 minutes, until softened and golden brown.

2. Meanwhile, make the Yorkshire puddings. Pour the sunflower oil into four muffin cups. When you turn the roasting veggies, place the muffin pan in the oven to heat up for 10 minutes. You want it to be really hot when you add the batter.

3. While the oil is heating, place the flour, soy milk, eggs, and spinach in a food processor and blend until well blended, about 1 minute. Then stir in the poppy seeds.

4. Carefully remove the muffin pan from the oven and pour in the batter. Place the pan right back in the oven and bake for 20 to 25 minutes, until the puddings have risen and are slightly golden on top. Don't open the oven door, as it will prevent them from rising.

5. Remove the Yorkshires from the oven. If the veggies aren't quite done, add the whole grains, nuts, and seeds and cook for 5 minutes, until lightly toasted. If the veggies are ready, transfer to a plate and cover with foil. Spread the whole grains, nuts, and seeds on the heated baking sheet, and bake for 5 minutes.

6. Divide the roasted veggies, toppings, and Yorkshire puddings among the plates. Pour on the gravy.

Switch Prefer a "naked," aka gravy-free, roast? Cover your veggies in one of these flavor options before roasting: 1 tablespoon rosemary, 1 tablespoon thyme, and 1 to 2 teaspoons za'atar or 1 teaspoon smoked paprika, and a big pinch of salt and black pepper.

Storage The leftover roasted veggies will keep in the fridge for 3 days, but I suggest using it up in my Reinvented Couscous Salad recipe (page 210). Cooked Yorkshires can be frozen for up to 1 month in an airtight container. The gravy will keep in the fridge for 3 days or can be frozen for up to 1 month.

Barley Butternut Risotto

Plant Points 6.75

Serves **4**   Prep **10 minutes**   Cook **40 minutes**

 Fridge Raid   **Freezer**

There are few things more comforting than a bowl of creamy risotto. Switching up the whole grain from rice to barley gives it a deliciously nutty taste (not to mention the added fiber—13 grams per portion)—and you can mix up the other plants depending on what's in season or what you have in the fridge.

2 tablespoons extra virgin olive oil
½ butternut squash or sweet
    potato, diced
1 leek, sliced
3 celery stalks, sliced
3 garlic cloves, grated or crushed
8 sage leaves or ½ teaspoon dried sage
1¼ cups (250 g) pearl barley
3¾ cups (900 ml) vegetable stock
1 ounce (30 g) Parmesan, grated
5 cups (150 g) mixed greens or
    spinach, chopped
Sea salt
Fresh ground black pepper

To Serve (optional)
Extra virgin olive oil, for frying
4 sage leaves
2 tablespoons pumpkin seeds
0.75 ounce (20 g) Parmesan, shaved
Lemon zest, to taste

1. Heat the olive oil in a large Dutch oven or saucepan over medium heat. Add the squash, leek, and celery and cook, stirring occasionally, until the vegetables start to soften, 10 minutes.

2. Stir in the garlic and sage, and cook until fragrant, 1 minute, then add adding the barley followed by the vegetable stock. Bring up to a gentle boil and cook, stirring occasionally, until the barley is al dente, 30 minutes. Add a splash of water if it gets too dry.

3. Stir in the grated Parmesan, followed by the greens. Cook until the greens are just wilted, about 3 to 4 minutes. Season to taste.

4. Serve with some crispy sage leaves and pumpkin seeds (if desired). Heat a splash of olive oil in a frying pan over medium-high heat, then drop in the sage leaves and pumpkin seeds and fry until crisp, 1 minute. You can also serve with Parmesan shavings and lemon zest.

Storage This risotto can be kept in the fridge for 3 days or frozen (minus the greens) for up to 1 month.

Switch To make this 100 percent plant-based, simply switch the Parmesan out for 2 tablespoons nutritional yeast or more to taste.

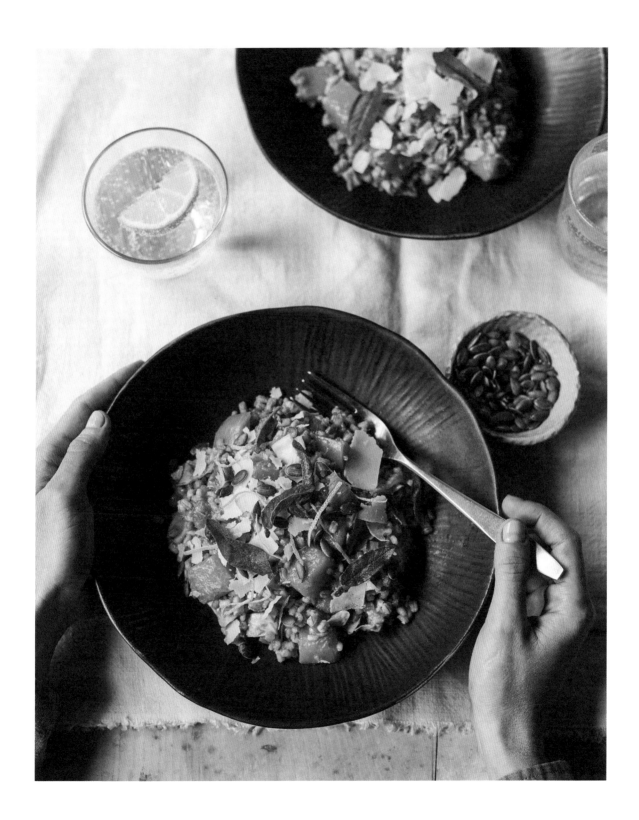

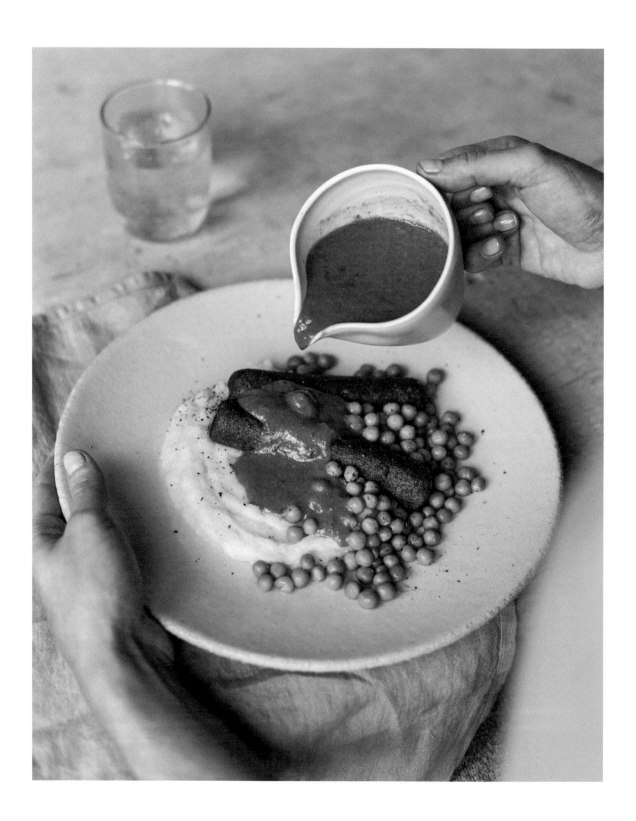

Bangers and Mash, Revamped

Plant Points
7.75

Serves **4**   Prep **15 minutes**   Chill **10 minutes**   Cook **20 minutes**

 Freezer

A plant-powered twist on a classic British dish. Creamy prebiotic vegetable mash topped with meaty plant-sausages and fresh green peas and drizzled with mouth-watering gravy—this recipe will be a family favorite.

2 to 3 slices seeded bread (about 3.5 ounces/100 g)

2 tablespoons flaxseed meal

1 large eggplant (about 14 ounces/ 400 g), roughly chopped

4 ounces (115 g) button mushrooms or mushrooms of choice, roughly chopped

1 apple, roughly chopped

3 tablespoons extra virgin olive oil

2 tablespoons Worcestershire sauce

1 tablespoon dried oregano

Sea salt

Fresh ground black pepper

Half of a 15-ounce (425 g) can green lentils, drained and rinsed

½ cup (15 g) finely chopped parsley

To Serve

2 heaping cups (320 g) peas, fresh or frozen

Vegetable Mash with Wild Mushroom Gravy (page 272)

1. To make the sausages, place the bread and flaxseed in a food processor and blend to form a coarse flour, 30 to 45 seconds. Transfer to a bowl, then set aside. Place the eggplant, apple, and mushrooms in the food processor and pulse until roughly chopped.

2. Heat 1 tablespoon of olive oil in a frying pan over medium-high heat, and add the eggplant mixture along with the Worcestershire sauce and oregano. Cook until the liquid from the veggies has reduced and the mixture has softened, about 10 minutes. Season to taste, then transfer to the food processor with the bread mixture. Add the lentils and parsley. Blend to form a rough mixture, 30 seconds.

3. Chill the mixture in the fridge for at least 10 minutes to firm up while you prep the vegetable mash and gravy.

4. Divide the sausage mixture into ten equal portions. Roll each portion into a sausage shape. Heat 2 tablespoons of olive oil in the frying pan over low heat. Add the sausages and cook, turning gently until golden all over and heated through, 10 minutes.

5. Cook the peas following package instructions, and serve with the sausages, vegetable mash, and gravy.

Storage The uncooked sausage mixture will keep in the fridge for up to 2 days and can be frozen for up to 2 months.

Note The sausage mixture is also delicious when made into falafel-like patties and served in a pita with pickles and yogurt.

Chicken 'n' Veggie Meatballs

Plant Points
4.75

Serves **4 (makes 28 meatballs, with about 1 cup/230 g left over to make**

Reinvented Chicken Burgers)

Prep **15 minutes**   Cook **20 minutes**

 FODMAP-Lite   **Freezer**

All of the succulent chicken flavor with just half the meat, and a great way to introduce more veggies to a meat-loving palate. Versatility is the name of these juicy meatballs' game— you could bake and enjoy them with a salad or add them to a stir-fry or your favorite soup. But my favorite way to eat them is to drizzle them with hoisin sauce and serve them on a bed of fried quinoa (page 273). Plus, the leftover mixture can be turned into my Reinvented Chicken Burgers (page 207).

4 to 5 slices seeded bread or
  bread of choice
1 pound (450 g) boneless, skinless
  chicken thighs
0.5 ounce (15 g) ginger, peeled
  and sliced
1 teaspoon sea salt
1 green bell pepper, roughly chopped
1 carrot, roughly chopped
6 scallions, roughly chopped
1 cup (30 g) chopped fresh cilantro
1 large egg, beaten
Extra virgin olive oil, for drizzling
  and frying

1. Preheat the oven to 375°F (190°C). Line a baking sheet with parchment paper.

2. Place the bread in a food processor and pulse to form crumbs, about 15 seconds. Transfer to a bowl and set aside.

3. Place the chicken, ginger, and salt in the food processor and blend until smooth, about 1 minute. Add the pepper and carrot, and pulse about five times until the veggies are all finely chopped but still visible. You may need to scrape the sides down. Next, add the scallions and cilantro, and pulse a few times until chopped.

4. Add in the egg and bread crumbs, and pulse until just mixed. Set aside 8 ounces (230 g) for the burger recipe (if desired) and divide the rest into 28 small meatballs.

5. Spread the meatballs out on the baking sheet, drizzle with olive oil, and bake for 15 minutes, until cooked through. For golden brown meatballs, heat a layer of oil in a frying pan over medium heat and fry the meatballs for 5 minutes.

Storage The uncooked balls/burgers can be made 24 hours in advance and stored in the fridge ready to cook or frozen for up to 3 months in an airtight container. Defrost overnight and cook following the recipe instructions.

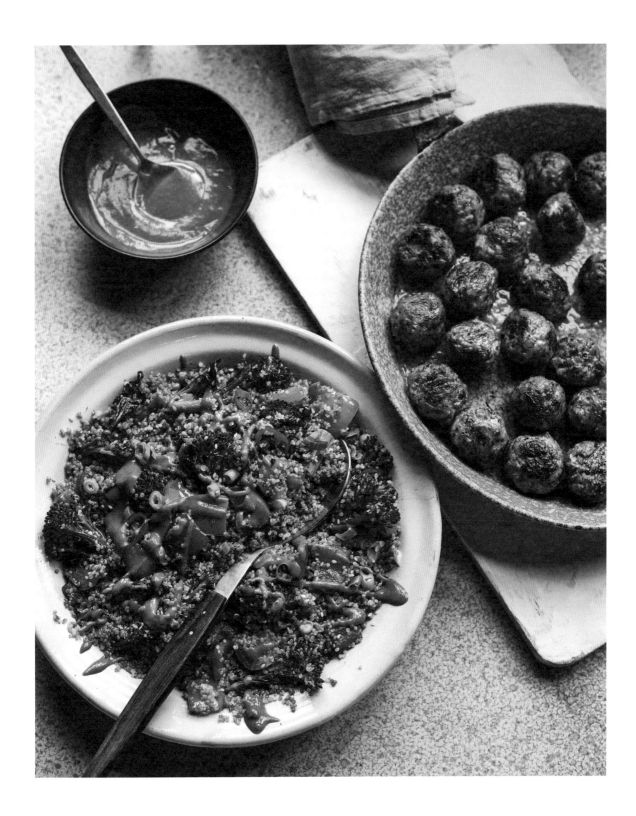

Sides

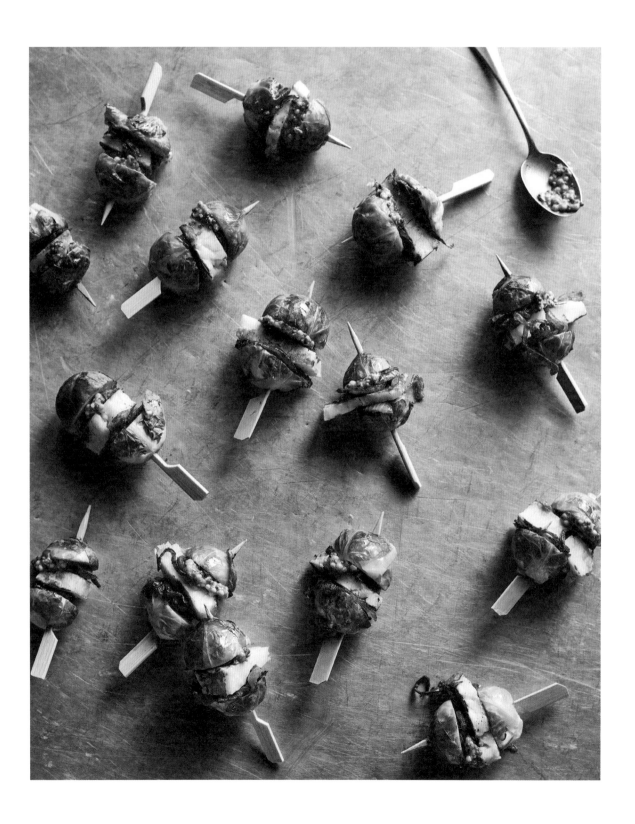

Halloumi Sprout Bites

Makes **15 bites**   Prep **20 minutes**   Cook **20 minutes**

If you're not big on Brussels sprouts, let me change your mind! Delicious roasted, the sweet-and-sour sticky onions and salty halloumi take them to the next level. Oh, and did you know sprouts and onions are both good sources of prebiotics, too?

15 large Brussels sprouts
1½ teaspoons extra virgin olive oil
3 ounces (85 g) halloumi, cut into
    5 slices
1 tablespoon whole grain mustard
Sea salt
Fresh ground black pepper

Caramelized Onions
1 tablespoon extra virgin olive oil
1 red onion, thinly sliced
1 tablespoon balsamic vinegar
1 Medjool date, made into a paste (see
    page 136), or 1 tablespoon sweetener

Cocktail sticks

1. Preheat the oven to 400°F (200°C). Line a baking sheet with parchment paper.

2. Place the sprouts in a medium bowl, then toss with olive oil, salt, and pepper. Spread out on the baking sheet and bake for 12 to 15 minutes, until just cooked and starting to take on a little color.

3. Meanwhile, make the caramelized onions. In a medium frying pan, heat 1 tablespoon of olive oil over medium heat, then add the onion, balsamic vinegar, and date paste. Cook, stirring frequently, until sticky and caramelized, at least 15 minutes.

4. In a small frying pan over medium heat, fry the halloumi until golden, 1 to 2 minutes on each side. Remove from the pan and set aside.

5. To assemble, cut each slice of halloumi into three pieces. Cut each sprout in half. Place one half on a cocktail stick, add some onion, and hold in place with a piece of halloumi. Add a little more onion and a little drop of mustard, then top with the other half of the sprout. Repeat until all are assembled, and enjoy!

Storage This will keep for 3 days in the fridge.

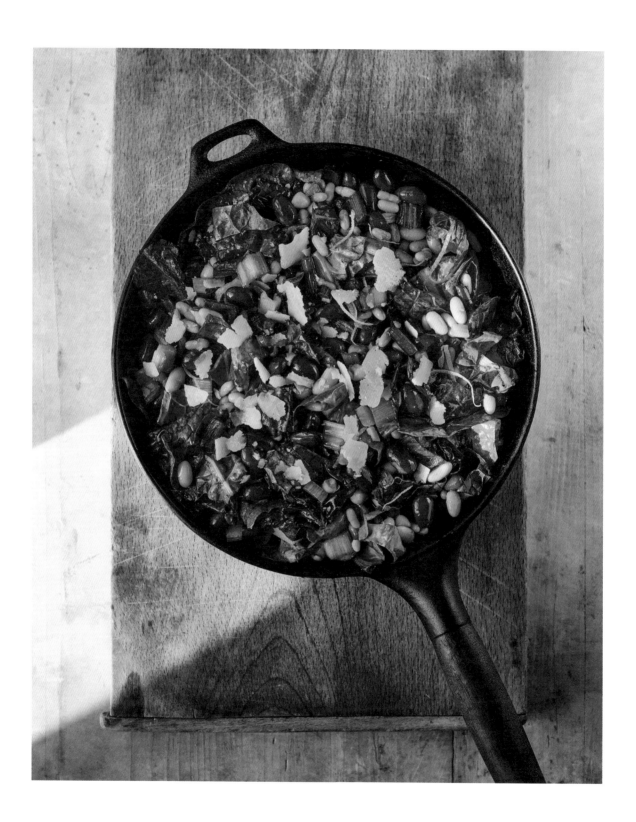

Greens and Beans

Plant Points
3.5

Serves **6**   Prep **5 minutes**   Cook **5 minutes**

 FODMAP-Lite   **Fridge Raid**   **Zero Waste**

My top fiber and diversity tip: Add a side of veggies or beans to whatever you're having (including your Saturday night takeout!). This quick and easy dish is the ideal way to do just that, packing in 10 grams of fiber per portion. It's the perfect example of how a little seasoning and light cooking can transform a humble can of beans and greens into a stunningly simple but tasty side in 10 minutes flat.

2 tablespoons extra virgin olive oil

2 garlic cloves, grated

10.5 ounces (300 g) Swiss chard, stems finely chopped and leaves roughly chopped, or greens of choice (e.g., bok choy, spinach, collard greens)

One 15-ounce (425 g) can cannellini beans, drained and rinsed

One 15-ounce (425 g) can red kidney beans, drained and rinsed

Zest of 1 lemon, or to taste

1½ teaspoons soy sauce

1.5 ounces (40 g) Parmesan, grated

Heat the olive oil and garlic in a large frying pan over medium heat for 1 minute, then add the greens. Saute until wilted, 2 minutes, then add the beans, lemon zest, and soy sauce. Serve straight out of the pan with some grated Parmesan.

Switch Up for the diversity challenge? Swap the greens for a package of mixed stir-fry vegetables.

Sticky Parsnips

Plant Points
5.5

Serves **4**   Prep **5 minutes**   Cook **15 minutes**

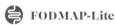 **FODMAP-Lite**

Not a fan of parsnips? Neither was I, until I discovered I just wasn't dressing them right. The sticky marinade in this recipe really elevates the humble parsnip. And it gets even better for busy people as the marinade has a dual role, coating the parsnips and marinating the Orange-Glazed Roasted Salmon on page 228.

1½ pounds (750 g) parsnips
Sesame oil, for frying

Marinade
Juice of 1 orange (about ⅓ cup/80 ml)
3 tablespoons mirin
3 tablespoons soy sauce
2 Medjool dates, made into a paste (see page 136), or 2 tablespoons sweetener
1 tablespoon plus 1 teaspoon peeled, grated fresh ginger
2 garlic cloves, grated or minced
1 tablespoon sesame oil
1 tablespoon whole wheat flour, plus more for coating

To Serve (optional)
1 scallion, finely chopped
1 tablespoon sesame seeds

1. Top and tail the parsnips and cut into bite-size cubes. Steam on the stovetop for 10 minutes or microwave for 7 minutes with a splash of water.

2. Meanwhile, make the marinade. Place the orange juice, mirin, soy sauce, date paste, ginger, garlic, and sesame oil in a small saucepan, bring to a boil, then simmer until reduced and syrupy, 5 to 10 minutes. Remove from the heat and slowly sprinkle in the flour, stirring rapidly to prevent clumps from forming. Roll the parsnips in flour before coating with the thickened marinade.

3. Heat a layer of sesame oil in a frying pan over medium-high heat, then add the coated parsnips. Fry until golden brown, 1 to 2 minutes on each side. Keep your eye on them as they can burn easily.

4. Sprinkle with the scallions and sesame seeds if desired. These are best enjoyed hot from the pan.

Storage   This will keep in the fridge for up to 3 days.

Steamed Veggies All-Dressed-Up

Serves **4 as a side or 2 for a light meal**   Prep **10 minutes**   Cook **5 minutes**

 FODMAP-Lite   **Fridge Raid**

Gone are the days of forcing down boring veggies. This recipe shows how, with two simple dressing options, plain steamed vegetables can be transformed into a side you actually crave. These ones are served in a fun edible bowl that not just kids will love.

One 14-ounce (400 g) bag prepared
   mixed vegetables
4 small whole wheat wraps or wraps
   of choice

Avocado Pesto
½ ripe avocado
3 tablespoons extra virgin olive oil
2 tablespoons grated Parmesan or
   nutritional yeast
2 tablespoons pine nuts
⅓ cup (5 g) fresh basil
½ garlic clove
Sea salt
Fresh ground black pepper

Creamy Cashew Sauce
¼ cup (60 g) probiotic yogurt
⅓ cup (45 g) natural cashews
2 tablespoons extra virgin olive oil
Juice of ½ small lemon (about
   1 tablespoon)
1 teaspoon Dijon mustard
Sea salt
Fresh ground black pepper

1. Preheat the oven to 400°F (200°C). Turn a muffin pan over and tuck the wraps into the gaps to make diamond-shaped edible bowls. Bake in the oven for 5 minutes, until browned in spots, then set aside to cool.

2. Meanwhile, cook the mixed vegetables in the microwave according to package instructions (usually by piercing the bag and cooking for 3 to 4 minutes). Alternatively, open the package and steam the veggies over a saucepan of simmering water for 3 to 4 minutes.

3. To make the avocado pesto, put the avocado, olive oil, Parmesan, pine nuts, basil, and garlic in a bowl and blend with an immersion blender to make a thick sauce, about 2 minutes. Season to taste.

4. To make the creamy cashew sauce, put the yogurt, cashews, olive oil, lemon juice, and mustard in a small food processor and blend to make a thick sauce, about 2 minutes. If it's too thick to pour, add a splash of hot water to thin. Season to taste.

5. Assemble the veggies in the edible wrap, and dollop on the avocado pesto or creamy cashew sauce.

Storage   Both dressings will keep in the fridge for up to 3 days. I use the leftovers as dips, spreads, and even pasta sauce—they're so versatile!

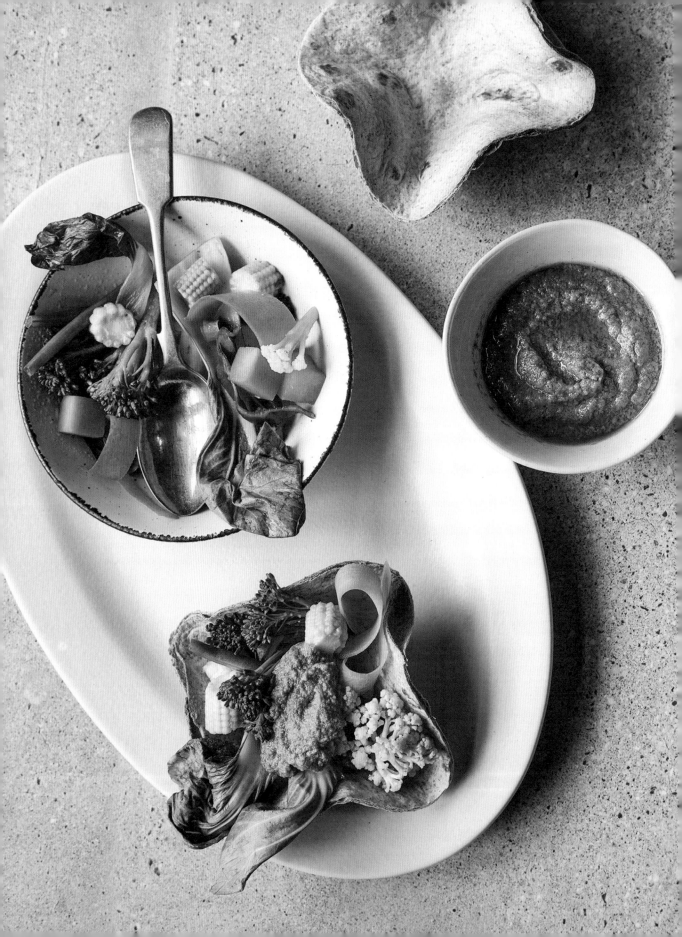

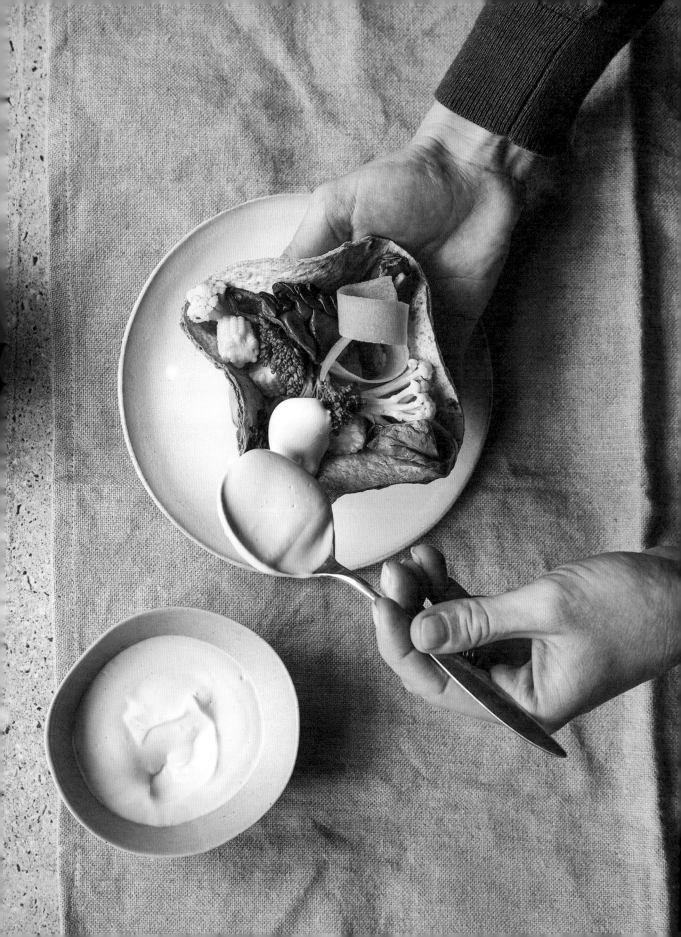

Spinach Balls with Tahini Sauce

Makes **20 bites**   Prep **15 minutes**   Cook **5 minutes**

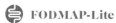 **FODMAP-Lite**

Inspired by the Japanese dish spinach gomae, this is a tasty way to get in your greens. These spinach balls are packed full of phytochemicals and fiber, and the tahini dipping sauce will have even those who aren't yet great with greens going back for more!

14 ounces (400 g) baby spinach

1 teaspoon sesame oil

1½ teaspoons tablespoon sesame seeds, toasted

Tahini Dipping Sauce

¼ cup (60 ml) tahini

Juice of 1 lemon (about 3 tablespoons), or to taste

2 Medjool dates, made into a paste (see page 136), or 2 tablespoons sweetener

1 teaspoon sesame oil

1 teaspoon soy sauce, or more to taste

Toothpicks

1. Place the spinach in a large saucepan over medium heat and cover. Allow to steam and wilt for 3 to 4 minutes. Rinse immediately under cold water and squeeze out any excess water, first with your hands and then in a clean cloth for the final squeeze. Place in a bowl and toss with the sesame oil.

2. To make the spinach balls, divide the spinach into 20 portions and shape into balls. Try to keep some of the leaves whole to wrap around each ball to hold it together. Place the balls on a kitchen or paper towel, to help absorb any excess liquid.

3. To make the dipping sauce, place the tahini, lemon juice, date paste, sesame oil, and soy sauce in a pitcher and blend with an immersion blender until smooth. Taste to check the balance of sweet, salty, and sour, adding a little more lemon juice or soy sauce as needed. If the sauce is a little thick, add a dash of water until it reaches your preferred consistency.

4. Transfer the spinach balls to a plate and scatter the sesame seeds on top. Serve with the dipping sauce and toothpicks.

Storage The spinach balls will keep for 2 days in the fridge. The tahini sauce will keep for up to 1 week in the fridge.

Tip If you can't find toasted sesame seeds, make your own. Heat a small nonstick frying pan over low heat. Add the sesame seeds and fry, stirring constantly, until lightly golden, 1 to 2 minutes.

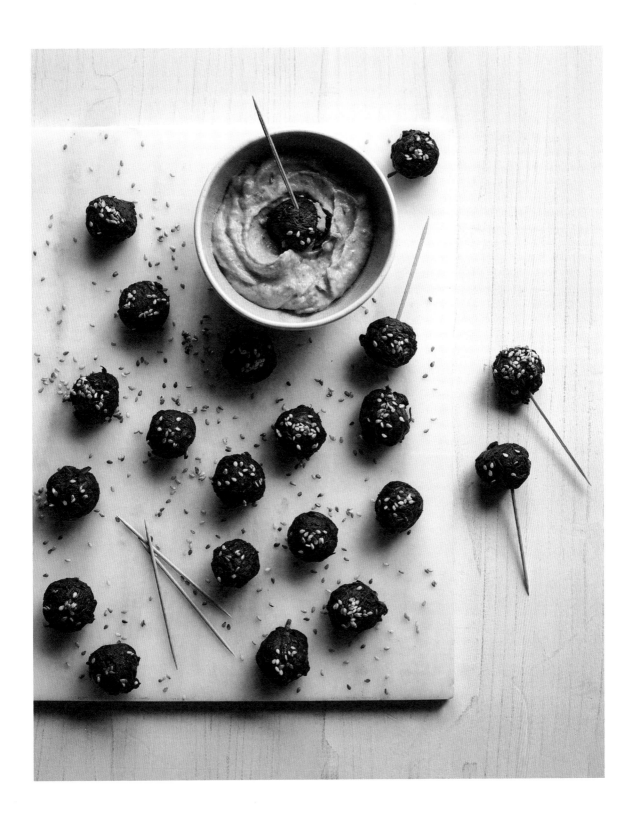

Vegetable Mash with Wild Mushroom Gravy

Plant Points
7.5

Serves **4**   Prep **15 minutes**   Cook **25 minutes**

 Freezer   **Zero Waste**

Gone are the days of single-plant-point mash. This smooth and fluffy potato, celeriac, and cauliflower mash, giving you triple plant points, is really brought to life with the wild mushroom gravy (pictured on page 256). A match made in mash heaven. Serve with bangers (Bangers and Mash, Revamped; page 257) or your protein of choice.

Creamy Mash

2 medium russet potatoes (about 1 pound/450 g), peeled and cut into 1.5-inch (4 cm) chunks

1 small celeriac, peeled and cut into 1 inch (2.5 cm) chunks

8 ounces (250 g) cauliflower florets

2 teaspoons extra virgin olive oil

½ cup (30 g) finely grated Parmesan, or more to taste

1 teaspoon Dijon mustard

Sea salt

Fresh ground black pepper

Wild Mushroom Gravy

2½ cups (600 ml) vegetable stock

0.5 ounce (15 g) dried porcini mushrooms

1 tablespoon olive oil

3.5 ounces (100 g) frozen sofrito vegetable mix (or 1 ounce/30 g each of carrot, onions, and celery, chopped)

2 tablespoons whole wheat flour or flour of choice

1 tablespoon red or white miso paste

1. To make the mash, bring a medium saucepan of water to a boil. Add the potato and celeriac and cook for 10 minutes. Add the cauliflower and cook until soft, 5 to 10 minutes. Drain and leave to dry for a few minutes, while you make the gravy.

2. To make the gravy, bring the vegetable stock to a boil, remove from the heat, then add the dried mushrooms. Allow to soak for 15 minutes.

3. Once the veggies have cooled, blend with an immersion blender until smooth, about 1 minute. Return the saucepan to a low heat and cook, stirring frequently, to simmer off any liquid from the veggies, 5 minutes. Take off the heat before stirring in the olive oil, Parmesan, and mustard. Season to taste, then cover to keep warm.

4. Heat the olive oil for the gravy in a frying pan over medium heat. Add the sofrito mix and cook until softened and starting to take on some color, 5 minutes.

5. Strain the stock, remove the mushrooms, and add the stock to a blender, along with the sofrito, flour, and miso paste. Blend until smooth, about 1 minute.

6. Return the gravy to the pan and simmer until thickened, stirring regularly, 10 minutes.

Storage The gravy freezes well for up to 3 months, so you could double the quantity and freeze half. It will keep in the fridge for up to 3 days.

Tip Love a chunky gravy? Keep half of the mushrooms when you strain the stock and blend. Add any leftover mushrooms to your next stir-fry. Don't throw them out!

Fried Quinoa with Hoisin Drizzle

Plant Points
7.75

Serves **4**   Prep **10 minutes**   Cook **7 minutes**

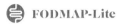 **FODMAP-Lite**

When you taste this flavorful and fiber-filled rice alternative, you'll wonder why you hadn't tried this rice-alternative sooner. **Not only does it add more texture, but it soaks up the sweet and salty hoisin drizzle perfectly (pictured on page 259). Enjoy it with Chicken 'n' Veggie Meatballs (page 258).**

Hoisin Drizzle
¼ cup (60 ml) soy sauce
2 tablespoons peanut butter
1 Medjool date, made into a paste (see page 136), or 1 tablespoon sweetener
2 teaspoons sesame oil
1 teaspoon balsamic vinegar
1 small garlic clove, grated or minced
½ teaspoon red miso paste

1½ teaspoons extra virgin olive oil
2 bell peppers, diced
3.5 ounces (100 g) Broccolini, chopped
1 large red chile, sliced
2¼ cups (405 g) cooked quinoa
Sea salt
Fresh ground black pepper
2 scallions, sliced
2 teaspoons sesame seeds (optional)

1. To make the hoisin drizzle, place the soy sauce, peanut butter, date paste, sesame oil, balsamic vinegar, garlic, and miso paste in a high-speed blender and blend until smooth.

2. Heat the olive oil in a large frying pan or wok. Add the peppers, Broccolini, and chile, and cook until just starting to take on some color, 3 to 4 minutes.

3. Add the quinoa and season to taste. Cook until the quinoa is heated through, 2 to 3 minutes, then stir in the scallions and sesame seeds (if using).

4. Drizzle the sauce over the quinoa and serve.

Note For added diversity, choose a multicolored pack of peppers. This dish also works well with red rice, for an extra plant point and hit of phytochemicals.

Storage Leftover hoisin drizzle will keep in a jar for up to 2 weeks in the fridge.

Desserts

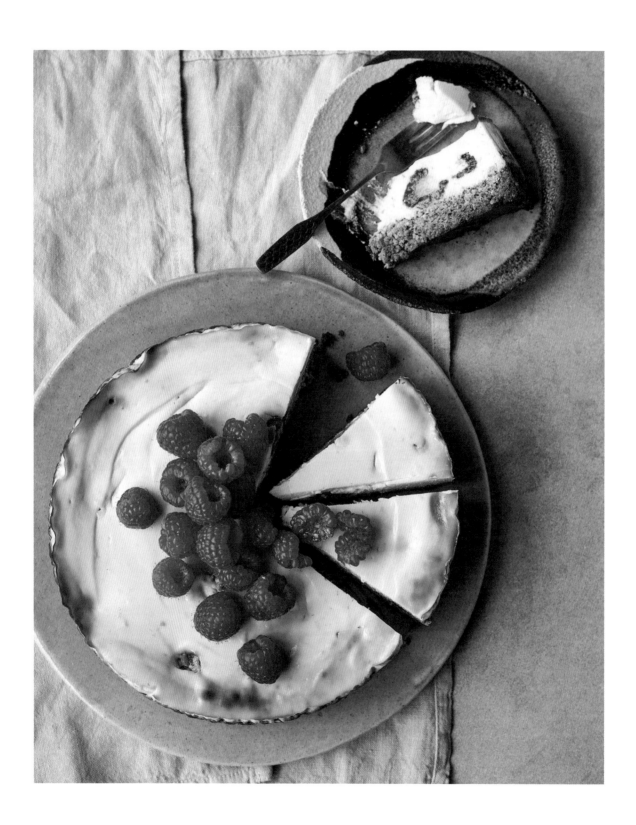

Raspberry and Lemon Ricotta Cheesecake

Makes **12 slices**   Prep **15 minutes**   Cook **1 hour**   Chill **8 hours**

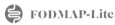 **FODMAP-Lite**

I love cheesecake, but store-bought versions can be notoriously high in saturated fat. This creamy cheesecake is a gut-loving treat, with fermented dairy, bursts of color from the juicy berries, and a deliciously nutty base that's just sweet enough.

Crust
2 cups (200 g) walnuts
½ cup (90 g) cooked quinoa
6 Medjool dates, pitted
1 tablespoon ground ginger (optional)
1 large egg, lightly beaten

Cheesecake
2 cups (500 g) ricotta
Generous ¾ cup (200 g) probiotic
   yogurt
2 large eggs, plus 1 egg yolk (use the
   leftover white to make an Omelet
   Bowl, page 141)
3 tablespoons all-purpose flour
3 tablespoons honey, or sweetener
   of choice
Juice of 1 lemon (about 3 tablespoons),
   plus zest to taste
1 cup (150 g) frozen raspberries

To Serve
⅔ cup (100 g) fresh raspberries

1. Preheat the oven to 375°F (190°C) and line the base and sides of a 9-inch (23 cm) springform pan with parchment paper.

2. To make the crust, place the walnuts, quinoa, dates, and ground ginger in a food processor and blend until combined (30 to 60 seconds), leaving some texture in the crumb. Stir in the egg.

3. Transfer to the cake pan and press down in an even layer. Bake for 20 minutes, until golden brown.

4. While the crust bakes, make the cheesecake. Place the ricotta, yogurt, eggs and egg yolk, flour, and honey in a food processor and blend to combine, about 1 minute. Scrape the sides and blend again for another minute.

5. When the crust has baked for 20 minutes, take it out and pour the cheesecake mixture on top, dotting in the frozen berries as you go.

6. Lower the oven to 350°F (180°C) and return the cake pan to the oven. Bake for 40 minutes, until the middle has just set. If there's still any wobble, give it another 5 to 10 minutes.

7. Turn the oven off, crack the door open and allow the cake to cool in the oven. Then remove and chill in the fridge overnight before serving with fresh berries.

Storage This is best eaten soon after it's chilled but will keep up to 5 days in an airtight container in the fridge.

Switch Already had raspberries this week? Swap for blueberries.

Trail Mix Loaf Cake with Yogurt and White Chocolate Glaze

Plant Points
10

Makes **12 slices**   Prep **15 minutes**   Cook **40 minutes**

 FODMAP-Lite   **Freezer**

My gut-loving take on a traditional fruit cake. Not only is it quick and easy to make for those on a tight schedule, but unlike boring fruit cakes, the diverse mix of textures and flavors will have you going back for seconds. It's ideal as an afternoon treat to share with friends and family, or you can drop the glaze and have it as a snack on the go to fuel those busy days.

4 very ripe bananas
3 large eggs
1 teaspoon vanilla extract
1⅓ cup (200 g) whole wheat flour
2 teaspoons baking powder
1 raw beet (about 3.5 ounces/100 g), coarsely grated
1 cup (100 g) walnuts, roughly chopped
8 dried figs (about 2.5 ounces/70 g), roughly chopped
⅓ cup (45 g) almonds, chopped
⅓ cup (50 g) dried mango, chopped
1 tablespoon mixed seeds

Glaze
3.5 ounces (100 g) white chocolate
¼ cup (60 g) probiotic yogurt

1. Preheat the oven to 375°F (190°C) and line a 9 x 5-inch (23 x 13 cm) loaf pan with parchment paper.

2. Place the bananas, eggs, and vanilla extract in a food processor and blend until combined, about 1 minute.

3. Mix the flour and baking powder in a large bowl, then add the beet, walnuts, figs, almonds, mango, and seeds. Fold in the wet ingredients.

4. Pour the mixture into the pan and bake for 40 minutes or until a skewer comes out clean. Let cool in the pan on a wire rack, then remove the cake from the pan.

5. To make the glaze, melt the chocolate. Place the chocolate in a heatproof bowl and either place over a pan of simmering water to melt or heat in the microwave in 30-second bursts, stirring in between.

6. Mix the yogurt into the melted chocolate, then spread over the cake.

Storage The cake (without the glaze) can be kept in an airtight container in the fridge for 5 days. It can also be frozen, wrapped in plastic wrap, for up to 1 month.

Cream-less Ice Cream, Two Ways

 FODMAP-Lite   Freezer

Whose freezer wouldn't benefit from a tub of gut-loving ice cream? You certainly don't need a special ice-cream machine—or even cream or added sugar—to make an indulgent and smooth dessert. If you love experimenting (or encouraging the kids to eat their greens!), the hidden-veggie version is for you; and if you're short on time, jump straight to the no-freeze option.

Hidden-Veggie Ice Cream

Serves **4**   Prep **15 minutes**   Freeze **4 hours**   Cook **2 minutes (if using cabbage)**

1 cup (70 g) shredded cabbage (optional)

2 large very ripe bananas, roughly chopped and frozen

Half of a 13.5-ounce (398 ml) can full-fat coconut milk, frozen

½ avocado

3 Medjool dates, pitted and roughly chopped

⅓ cup (10 g) baby spinach

Optional Fillings (choose one)

2 tablespoons mint leaves and ⅓ cup (50 g) dark chocolate chips, roughly chopped

13.5 ounces (100 g) Prebiotic Cookie Dough Drops (page 165)

1. To steam the cabbage (if using), fill a steamer with 1 inch (2.5 cm) of water and bring to a boil. Place the cabbage in the basket, cover and steam until soft, 5 minutes. Alternatively, add a little water to a microwave-safe dish and microwave for 2 minutes on high or until the cabbage has softened. Place in the freezer to chill completely.

2. Take the bananas and coconut milk out of the freezer 5 minutes before you want to make the ice cream; this will make it easier to blend. Cut the frozen coconut milk into small chunks and place them in a high-powered blender along with the banana. Blend until the ice crystals have broken down (it will look like slushy snow), 5 minutes.

3. Add the avocado, cabbage (if using), dates, and spinach. Blend until smooth, 4 to 5 minutes. You may need to stop and scrape down the sides occasionally.

4. If using fillings, blend the mint through the ice cream for a few seconds and stir through the chocolate chips, or stir in chunks of the cookie dough.

5. Pour the ice cream into a 1-quart (1 L) airtight tub as quickly as you can, to limit melting, and place it in the freezer for at least 4 hours to firm up.

No-Freeze Ice Cream

Serves **4**   Prep **5 minutes**

3 cups (420 g) frozen
    blueberries or berry
    of choice
Generous 1½ cups (400 g)
    probiotic yogurt
2 very ripe bananas, frozen

Place the berries, yogurt, and bananas in a high-powered blender and blend until smooth, about 1 minute—and you're done! Serve and enjoy.

Storage This can be frozen in an airtight container for up to 1 month.

Tip Chill the tub in the freezer while you're making the ice cream so it's cold when you pour the ice cream in. This will help prevent the mixture from melting, which will result in a creamier ice cream.

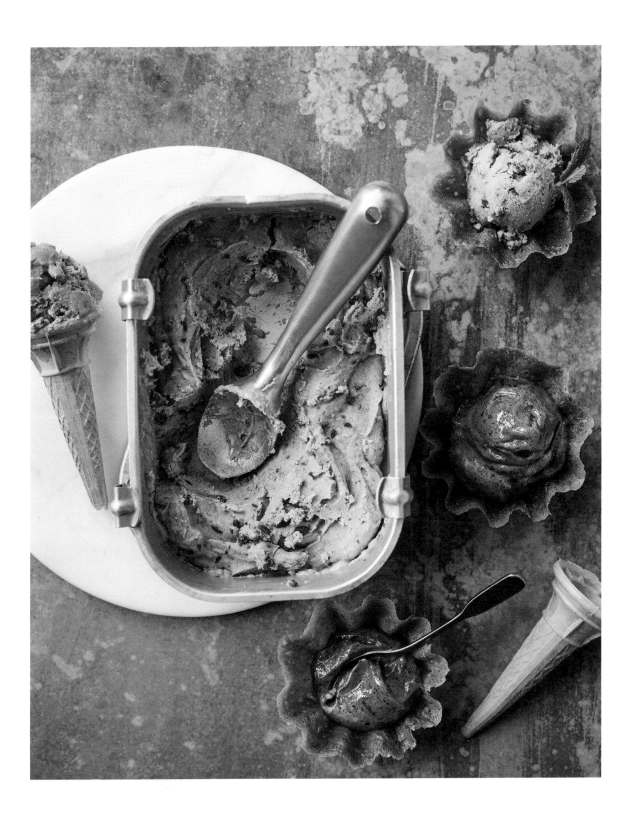

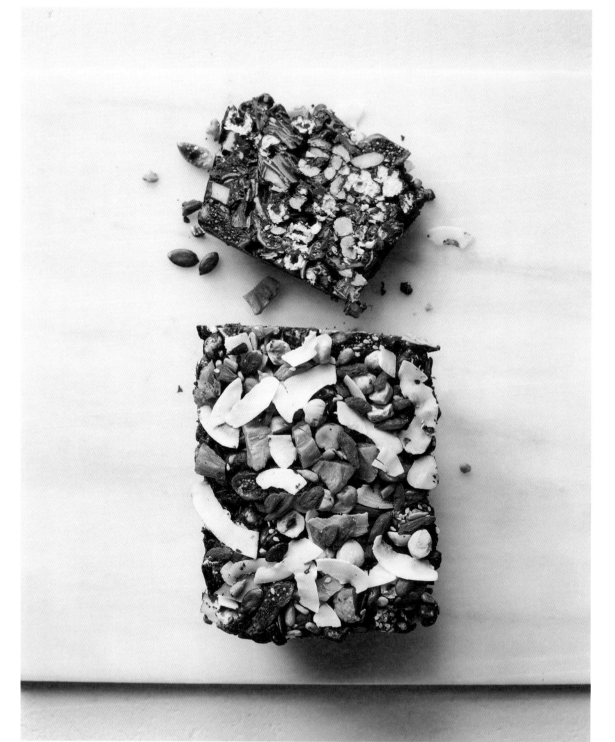

Prebiotic Rocky Road

Plant Points **10.5**

Makes **15 slices**   Prep **15 minutes**   Chill **4 hours**   Cook **5 minutes**

🔄 **FODMAP-Lite**   ♻ **Zero Waste**

With the combination of melt-in-your-mouth chocolate, crunchy nuts, chewy fruit, and fluffy popcorn, this gut-loving treat trumps your standard rocky road on flavor. Your gut microbes will get quite the feast of phytochemicals, prebiotics, and 5 grams of fiber per slice, using only pantry ingredients. Plus, the cocoa flavanols in dark chocolate could even boost your brain power!

10.5 ounces (300 g) dark chocolate (at least 70 percent)
1 tablespoon extra virgin olive oil, plus extra for popping corn
¾ cup plus 2 tablespoons (100 g) hazelnuts, chopped in half
2½ tablespoons popcorn kernels
10 dried figs (about 3 ounces/ 90 g), chopped
3 ounces (85 g) dried mango, chopped
⅓ cup (45 g) Brazil nuts, roughly chopped
½ cup (50 g) dried goji berries
½ cup (30 g) coconut flakes
2 tablespoons mixed seeds

1. Toast the hazelnuts. Heat the oven to 400°F (200°C) and place the nuts on a baking sheet. Bake for 5 minutes, then remove and set aside to cool.

2. To pop the corn, heat a splash of olive oil in a saucepan over medium heat. Add the popcorn kernels and shake gently to cover them in the oil, then cover the pan. The corn will start popping after a few minutes. Shake the saucepan occasionally to prevent burning. The corn will finish popping after 3 to 5 minutes.

3. Pour the popcorn into a large bowl and mix with the hazelnuts, figs, mango, Brazil nuts, goji berries, coconut flakes, and seeds, reserving a handful of the ingredients to decorate the top of the rocky road.

4. Break the chocolate into pieces and place in a heatproof bowl. Place over a saucepan of simmering water to melt or heat in the microwave in 30-second bursts, stirring in between. Stir in 1 tablespoon of olive oil, before pouring over the dry ingredients and mixing everything together well.

5. Line a 9 x 5-inch (23 x 13 cm) loaf pan with parchment paper, then pour the mixture into the pan. Scatter the reserved dry ingredients on top and press down. Place in the fridge to set, about 4 hours.

6. Once set, pull the rocky road out of the pan using the parchment paper, cut into 15 slices, and store in an airtight container in the fridge.

Storage This will keep for up to 2 weeks in the fridge in a sealed container.

Tip If you love ginger, add ¼ to ½ teaspoon of fresh grated ginger to the mixture.

Switch Already had these dried fruits and nuts this week? Swap in any others you like.

Pistachio Berry Bursts

Makes **40 pieces**   Prep **25 minutes**   Chill **30 minutes**

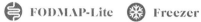 **FODMAP-Lite**   ✳ **Freezer**

I must say, I'm quite proud of this one. It combines three of my favorite things: prebiotic pistachios, raspberries, and white chocolate, all packed into little bursts of joy—and I'd argue even more aesthetically pleasing than your standard box of chocolates. Want to impress a friend (and their gut microbes)? Make these!

⅔ cup (80 g) pistachios
1 teaspoon extra virgin olive oil
½ teaspoon vanilla extract
3 ounces (85 g) white chocolate
40 large raspberries (about
    1¼ cups/190 g)
3 ounces (85 g) dark chocolate
    (optional)

1. Place the pistachios, olive oil, and vanilla in a small food processor and blend until a paste forms, about 3 minutes. You may need to scrape down the sides occasionally. Transfer to a medium bowl.

2. Break the white chocolate into pieces and place in a heatproof bowl. Place over a saucepan of simmering water to melt or heat in the microwave in 30-second bursts, stirring in between. Pour into the bowl with the pistachios and mix to form a dough.

3. Fill each raspberry with the mixture, using clean fingers or a piping bag, so that the tops of the raspberries are domed with the filling. Place in the fridge for a few minutes to set.

4. Meanwhile, break the dark chocolate (if using) into pieces and melt.

5. Line a baking sheet with parchment paper, then carefully dip each filled raspberry in the melted chocolate using 2 teaspoons or just your fingers. You can dip just the domed pistachio top, like an ice cream, completely cover them, or do a mix of both.

6. Place on the baking sheet, then place in the fridge to set, 30 minutes, before digging in.

Storage The filled raspberries will keep for 3 days in the fridge or up to 1 month in the freezer, although I doubt they'll last that long. The pistachio filling on its own will keep for a couple of weeks in a small sealed jar in the fridge and is delicious spread on apple or pear slices. Such a treat!

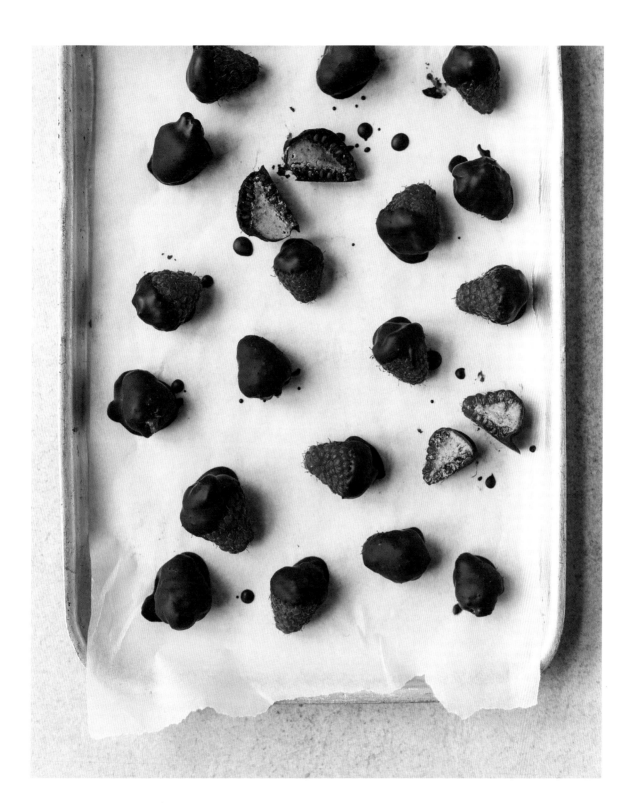

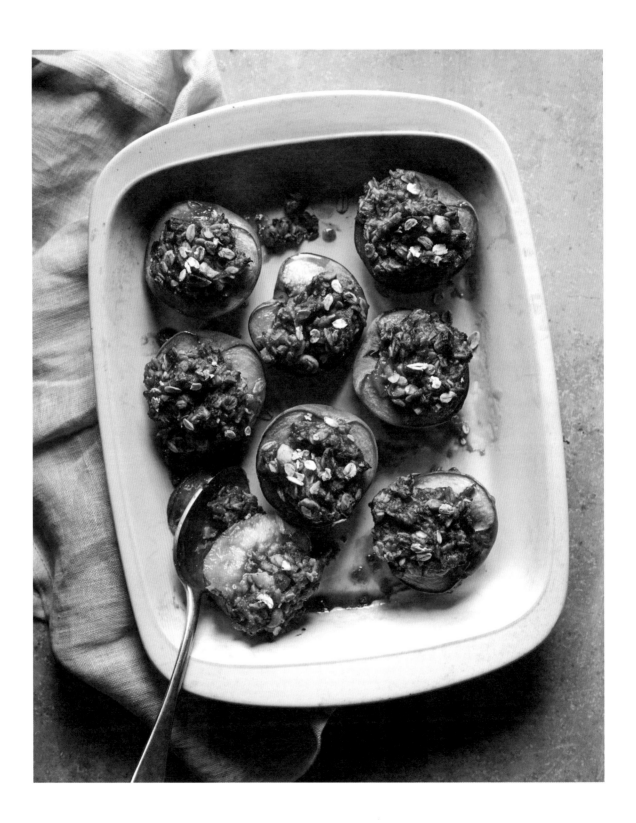

Naked Fruit Crumble

Plant Points
6.5

Serves **4**   Prep **10 minutes**   Cook **30 to 40 minutes (depending on the fruit)**

 Zero Waste

This comforting dessert brings back memories of digging into my granny's fruit crumble. I pop this in the oven as I sit down to dinner; by the time I've finished eating, the baked fruit, nut, and cinnamon aromas have filled the kitchen, and it's ready to eat. This recipe works all year round with whatever fruit is in season and contains double the fiber (not to mention the plant diversity) of a lone piece of fruit.

4 large extra ripe nectarines, peaches, apples, or pears, or a mix of each
6 Medjool dates, made into a paste (page 136), or 6 tablespoons sweetener of choice
1 tablespoon extra virgin olive oil
⅓ cup (35 g) mixed nuts, chopped
⅓ cup (35 g) rolled oats
½ teaspoon ground cinnamon
Juice of 1 lemon (about 3 tablespoons), plus zest to taste

To Serve
¼ cup (60 g) probiotic yogurt or Cream-less Ice Cream (page 279)

1. Preheat the oven to 375°F (190°C).

2. Cut the fruit in half (remove the core, if needed) and make a small hollow the size of a quarter. If using stone fruit, simply remove the pit.

3. Place the fruit, cut side up, in a small roasting pan. You want the fruit to sit snugly inside the pan, so it won't dry out. Set aside.

4. Mix the date paste, olive oil, and 1 tablespoon of water together in a medium bowl, then add the nuts, oats, cinnamon, and lemon juice. Mix to form a sticky crumble mixture. Taste and add zest to preference.

5. Fill the hollows of the fruit with equal amounts of the crumble.

6. Cover with foil and bake for 20 minutes for stone fruit or 30 minutes for apples or pears, then remove the foil and bake for 10 to 15 minutes more, until the crumble is golden brown and the fruit is tender.

7. Serve with your choice of yogurt or ice cream.

Tip Short on time? Cook the fruit in the microwave for 3 to 4 minutes first to soften it before adding the crumble and baking, uncovered, for 10 minutes or until golden brown.

Storage This is best served straight out of the oven. It will keep in the fridge for up to 3 days.

Switch Already had oats this week? Switch them for rye flakes.

Gut-Loving Carrot Cake with Vanilla Cream Frosting

Serves **12**   Prep **25 minutes, plus chilling**

 Zero Waste

This plant-packed cake is my raw and vegan version of a classic carrot cake—perfectly sweet, rich, and indulgent, it also nourishes your gut microbes. With each slice offering almost 6 grams of fiber, it's the perfect crowd-pleasing dessert to share with your foodie friends, and there are two toppings to choose from, depending on how much time you have on your hands.

18 Medjool dates, pitted and
   roughly chopped
1½ teaspoons ground cinnamon
½ teaspoon ground ginger
¼ teaspoon ground nutmeg
3 medium carrots, grated
2 cups (200 g) walnuts
1 cup (100 g) pecans
1 cup (100 g) almond meal
⅓ cup (50 g) raisins

Whipped Cream Topping
1 cup (240 ml) plant-based
   whipping cream
1 teaspoon vanilla extract
10 walnuts, crumbled

or

Coconut-Cashew Cream Topping
2¾ cups (355 g) cashews
1 cup (240 ml) coconut cream
¼ cup (60 ml) honey
Juice of ½ lemon (about
   1½ tablespoons), plus zest to taste
1 teaspoon vanilla extract

Storage This will keep in an airtight container in the fridge for 5 days.

Tip If you have any cake mixture left over, it's great for rolling into raw carrot cake snack balls!

1. Line a high-sided 9-inch (23 cm) cake pan with parchment paper on the base and sides, and set aside.

2. Place the dates, cinnamon, ginger and nutmeg in a food processor and blend until the mixture forms a ball, 1 to 2 minutes. Add the carrot and pulse to combine roughly, then transfer to a large bowl.

3. Blend the walnuts and pecans in the food processor and blend to form slightly chunky crumbs, about 20 seconds. Add to the bowl along with the almond meal and raisins. Use a wooden spoon to combine.

4. Transfer the batter to the pan and press down to compress and smooth the top. Chill in the fridge until you're ready to make the topping.

5. To make the whipped cream topping, whip the cream with the vanilla extract until it forms soft peaks, about 8 minutes. Spoon the cream onto the cake, sprinkle with the crumbled walnuts, and serve.

6. To make the alternative, more luxurious coconut-cashew cream topping, cover the cashews with boiling water and set aside to soak for at least 10 minutes. Strain the soaked cashews and place in a high-powered food processor along with the coconut cream, honey, lemon juice, lemon zest, and vanilla extract. Blend at high speed until super-smooth, 5 to 6 minutes, scraping down the sides occasionally. Pour over the carrot cake and smooth out the top. Place in the fridge to set for about 4 hours.

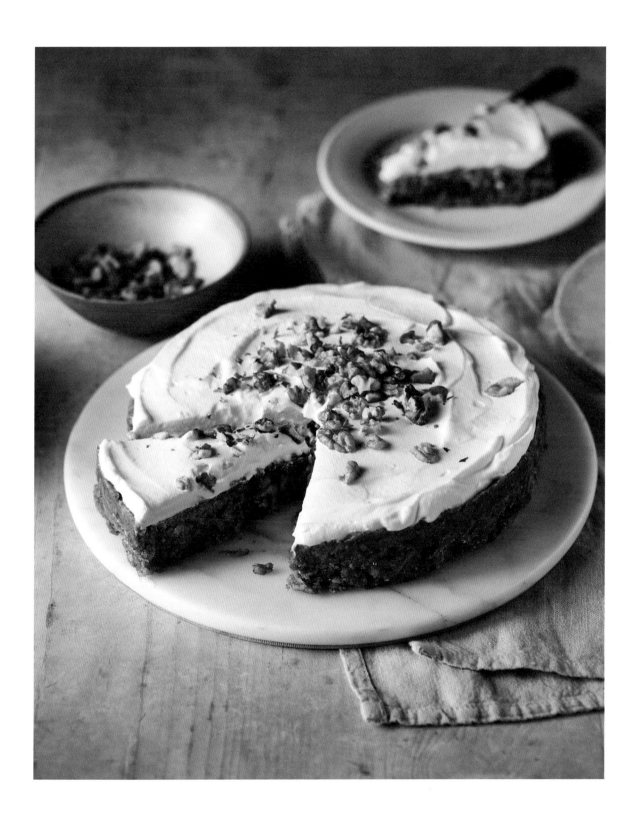

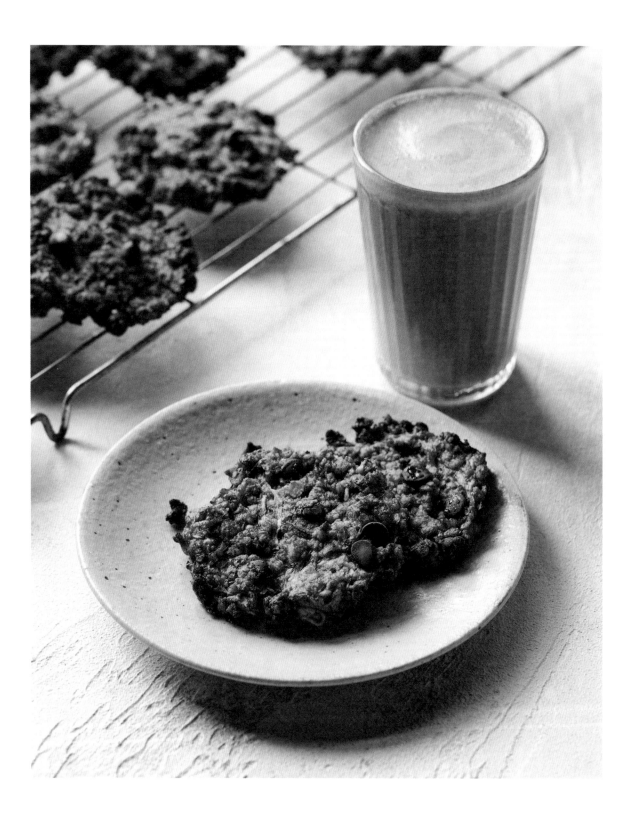

Chocolate Chip Zucchini Cookies

Makes **18 cookies**   Prep **15 minutes**   Cook **25 minutes**

 FODMAP-Lite   **Freezer**   **Zero Waste**

Combining the best of both worlds, these high-fiber chocolate chip cookies are a little crunchy and a little chewy, just like a good cookie should be. Plus, the hidden veggies give you an extra 4 plant points in one—and no one will ever know!

1 very ripe banana

6 Medjool dates, pitted and roughly chopped

1½ cups (150 g) rolled oats

¼ cup (60 ml) extra virgin olive oil, plus more for greasing

2 teaspoons vanilla extract

1 zucchini (about 5 ounces/140 g), grated

⅓ cup (50 g) dark chocolate chips or chocolate chips of choice

1. Preheat the oven to 350°F (180°C) and grease two baking sheets with olive oil.

2. Place the banana, dates, half the oats, the olive oil, and vanilla in a food processor and blend to form a paste, 1 minute.

3. Squeeze the grated zucchini in a clean cloth to remove the excess moisture, then place in a medium bowl. Add the chocolate chips, the remaining oats, and the banana-date mixture. Stir well to combine.

4. Spoon the mixture onto the baking sheets, making about 18 cookies, and gently smooth into flat rounds.

5. Bake for 25 to 30 minutes, until golden brown. Transfer to a wire rack and leave to cool completely.

Storage   These are best eaten fresh from the oven. They can be frozen baked or as raw dough for up to 1 month.

Drinks

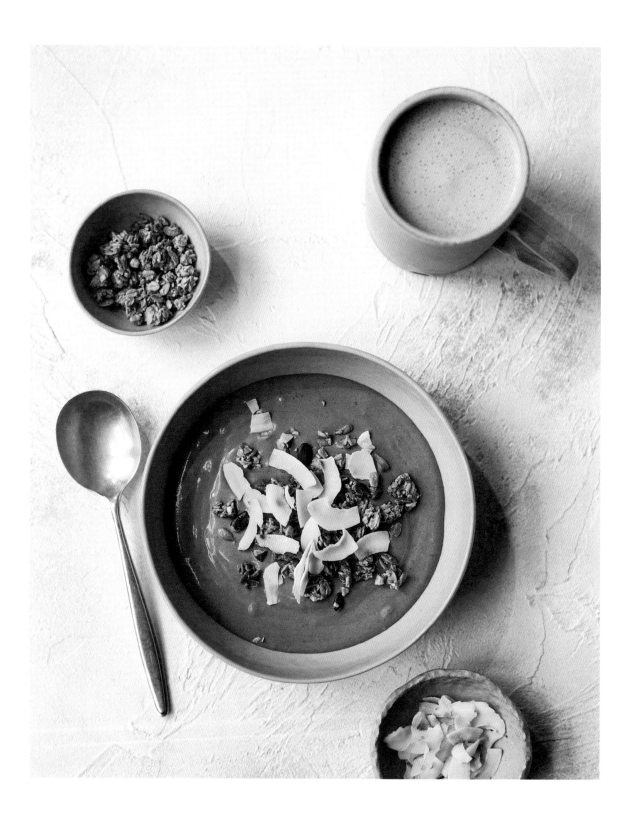

Snickers Smoothie Bowl

Serves **1 hungry person**   Prep **5 minutes**

 Freezer

Move over ultra-processed protein shakes: This bowl not only offers 18 grams of protein, 10 grams of fiber, and 6.25 plant points, but it tastes just like a Snickers chocolate bar— without the added sugar and additives.

1 very ripe banana, frozen
1.5 ounces (40 g) zucchini, frozen
2 ounces (55 g) silken tofu
¼ cup (60 g) probiotic yogurt
2 Medjool dates, pitted
1 tablespoon unsweetened cocoa powder
1 tablespoon nut butter of choice

Toppings (optional)
2 tablespoons no-sugar-added granola
   (see DIY Plant-Packed Granola,
   page 145)
2 tablespoons coconut flakes

1. Place the banana, zucchini, tofu, yogurt, dates, cocoa powder, and nut butter in a high-powered blender and blend until smooth, 1 minute.

2. Pour into a small bowl or cup and add your choice of toppings.

Switch Want a lighter option? Blend in 2.5 ounces (70 g) of ice with a little extra water to thin, and share with a friend. Alternatively, freeze the leftovers in an ice cube tray, and when you're ready for round two, blend together the frozen cubes and a little milk of choice. This will keep in the freezer for up to 1 month.

Tip If you add DIY Plant-Packed Granola (page 145), you'll get an extra 18.5 plant points.

Smoothies, Four Ways

Brain-Boosting Blueberry Smoothie

Plant Points **3**

Serves **1**   Prep **5 minutes**

 Zero Waste

Packed full of flavonoids shown to have brain-boosting properties, plus extra plant points and live microbes for good measure, this celebrates all the good that plants can do for our brain power.

¾ cup (105 g) frozen blueberries
2 frozen cauliflower florets
   (optional)
1 ripe pear, chopped
Generous ¾ cup (100 g)
   probiotic yogurt
Scant ½ cup (100 ml) water or milk
   of choice
Ice

Place the blueberries, cauliflower (if using), pear, yogurt, and water in a high-powered blender and blend until smooth. Serve over ice and enjoy.

Switch Want to up your plant points? Switch the blueberries for mixed berries.

Immunity-Nourishing Smoothie

Plant Points **4.5**

Serves **1**   Prep **5 minutes**

 FODMAP-Lite

Feeding your immune system while also satisfying your taste buds, this one is a bit of a no-brainer (remember, 70 percent of your immune cells live in your gut!). This is my go-to combo when winter strikes, but also when I'm craving something refreshing on a hot summer's day. This beauty serves up 10 grams of fiber—that's a third of your daily intake in one glass.

7 ice cubes
1 large orange, peeled and halved
1 carrot, halved
½ very ripe banana
¼ cup (25 g) walnuts
0.5 ounce (15 g) fresh ginger, peeled
⅓ cup (80 ml) soy milk or milk
   of choice
Big pinch of turmeric

Place the ice, orange, carrot, banana, walnuts, ginger, soy milk, and turmeric in a high-powered blender and blend until smooth, 1 minute. Taste and adjust the ginger, turmeric, and banana (for sweetness) to your preference.

Switch Had enough of carrots? Switch for 2.5 ounces (70 g) zucchini.

Greenie Crush

Plant Points
4.25

Serves **1**   Prep **5 minutes**

Creamy and refreshing, this smoothie packs **7** grams of fiber and **4** plant points. Your gut will thank you for making the switch from your fiber-stripped green juice.

5 ice cubes
1 apple, roughly chopped
½ cucumber, roughly chopped
1.75 ounces (50 g) silken tofu
¼ avocado
7 mint leaves, or more to taste
⅓ cup (80 ml) milk of choice

Place the ice, apple, cucumber, tofu, avocado, mint, and milk in a high-powered blender and blend until smooth, 1 minute. Taste and adjust the mint to your preference, and add additional milk, water, and/or ice to achieve your preferred consistency.

Switch No mint? Switch for 0.25 ounce (7 g) fresh ginger.

Raspberry Red

Plant Points
6

Serves **1**   Prep **5 minutes**

Forget those sickly sweet fruit-only smoothies—this combo is not only satisfyingly creamy but also offers plenty of plant-based diversity. A winning breakfast, snack or post-workout fuel, it has over **10** grams of fiber and **15** grams of protein per portion.

5 ice cubes, plus more to serve
½ cup (75 g) frozen raspberries
1 tablespoon dried cranberries or sweetener of choice
1 celery stalk
0.75 ounce (20 g) beet (optional)
¼ cup (20 g) rolled oats
⅓ cup (80 g) probiotic yogurt
1 tablespoon almond butter

Place the ice, raspberries, cranberries, celery, beet (if using), oats, yogurt, and almond butter in a high-powered blender along with ⅓ cup (80 ml) water and blend until smooth, 1 to 2 minutes. Taste and adjust the flavors to preference. Best served over ice.

Switch Love kefir? Me too! Swap the yogurt and water for ⅔ cup (160 ml) kefir.

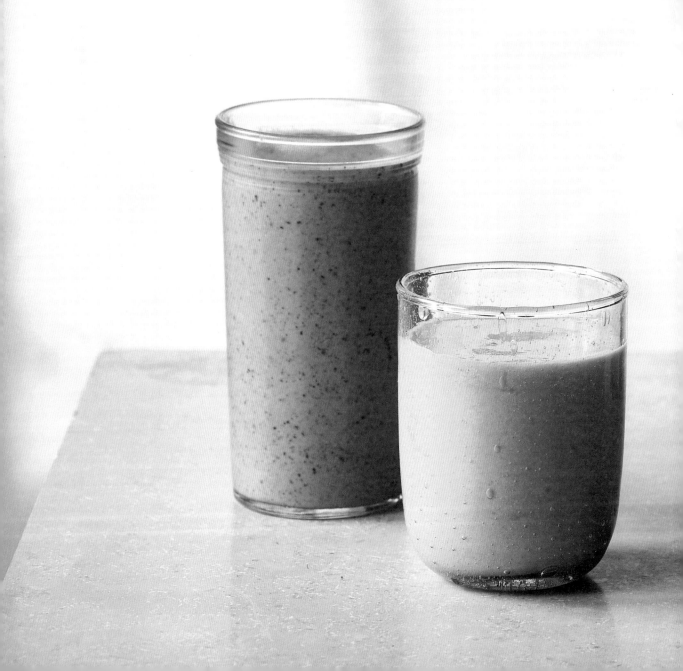

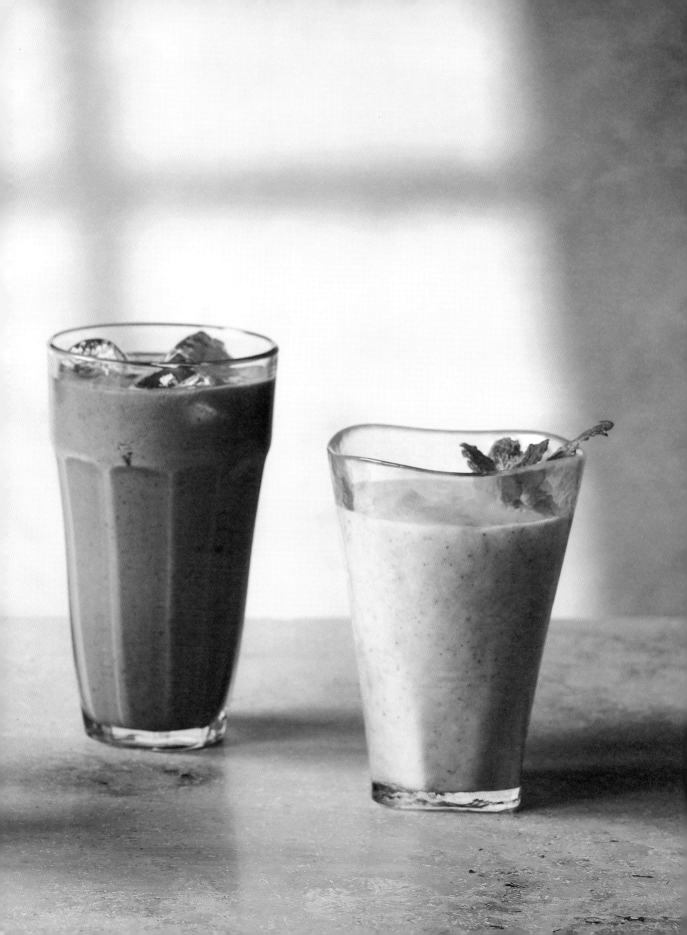

Microbe-Made Ginger Soda

Plant Points
0.25

Makes **Eight 1-cup (240 ml) servings** Prep **3 weeks (4 to 7 days for Ginger Bug;
10 to 14 days for Ginger Soda)**

FODMAP-Lite

Before machines, all sparkling drinks were microbe-made, so here's to bringing back the good old ways for a homemade refreshing fizz. If you want to experiment with the microbial world, but aren't quite ready for kefir or kombucha, then this is the recipe for you.

Step 1: Ginger Bug

2 teaspoons unpeeled grated
    fresh ginger, per day
2 teaspoons sugar, per day
1 cup (240 ml) filtered water

Equipment
One 16-ounce (or 500 ml)
    glass jar, sterilized
Clean cloth
Rubber band

1. Place the ginger, sugar, and water in the glass jar. Stir to dissolve the sugar, then cover with the cloth and secure with the rubber band.

2. Each day for the next 4 to 7 days, stir in an additional 2 teaspoons of ginger and 2 teaspoons of sugar (think of this as feeding the community of microbes). Give the jar a little swirl whenever you walk past it (aim for at least twice per day), to help evenly distribute the food to the microbes.

3. Depending on the climate (warmer temperatures will speed up the process; cooler ones will slow it down), by day 4 bubbles should start to appear in the jar (this is a sign the microbes are busy eating the sugar). Once the ginger has floated to the top of the jar and there are bubbles on the surface, your Ginger Bug is ready for graduation—you can move on to step 2.

Tip If there are no bubbles by day 7, it's best to ditch the batch and start again (there may not have been enough microbes in and on your ginger—try using organic ginger for the next batch if you haven't already).

Step 2: Ginger Soda

1¾ quarts (1.75 L) water (tap is fine, as you'll boil this)

Scant 1 cup (175 g) granulated or 1⅓ cups (175 g) unpacked brown sugar

2 to 4 tablespoon grated fresh ginger, to taste

1 cup (240 ml) strained Ginger Bug (from step 1)

Juice of 1 lemon (about 3 tablespoons)

Equipment

Two 1-quart (1 L) airtight glass bottles, sterilized

1. Bring the water, sugar, and ginger to a boil in a large covered saucepan for about 10 minutes. Taste and adjust the ginger to preferred flavor intensity. It will taste rather sweet, but rest assured that the microbes from your ginger bug will eat a lot of this sugar over the next 2 weeks.

2. Let cool completely, then add in the Ginger Bug and lemon juice and stir to combine. Decant the mix into the bottles, being sure to leave some headspace for the bubbles that the ginger bug will produce.

3. Seal the bottles and leave to ferment in a dark cupboard at room temperature for around 2 weeks (ideally between 65°F and 75°F/18°C and 24°C). Like the Ginger Bug, the warmer the temperature, the faster the microbes work, so be sure to adjust your timing accordingly. Every third day, open the lid to release the pressure and give it a little taste. You should notice the bubbles increasing over time as the sweetness settles.

4. Once it hits your preferred level of carbonation and sweetness, place it in the fridge (this will put the microbes to sleep) and, once chilled, enjoy a refreshing bubbly cup!

Storage This is best consumed within 2 weeks, although I doubt it'll last that long.

Frothy Cashew Latte

Plant Points
2.25

Serves **1**   Prep **5 minutes**

 FODMAP-Lite   **Zero Waste**

Forget all the soaking and straining: This nutty latte uses whole cashews, saving you time and giving you an extra hit of gut-loving prebiotic fiber. Did I mention it's deliciously creamy, too? A must-try!

1 cup (240 ml) hot coffee
¼ cup (30 g) roasted cashews
1 Medjool date

Place the coffee, cashews, and date in a high-powered blender and blend until smooth, 1 minute. Taste and adjust flavors to preference.

Tip For extra indulgence, use salted roasted cashews for a flavor explosion! While, yes, they contain a little added salt, in the grand scheme of the Diversity Diet, it's rather negligible.

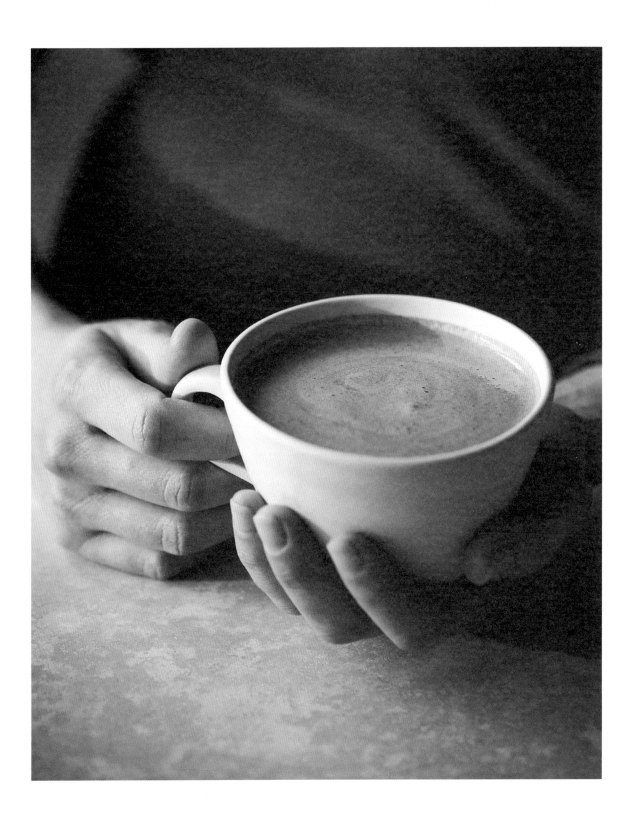

One-Minute Snacks

Sweet Potato Slider: Leftover cooked sweet potato with nut butter and a dollop of probiotic yogurt.

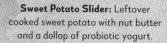 FODMAP-Lite

Prebiotic "Chocolate" Milkshake: Place 1 cup (240 ml) of your milk of choice, 2 Medjool dates, 1 tablespoon cocoa, 1 tablespoon nut butter of choice and ¼ teaspoon vanilla extract to a high-powered blender, and blend.

FODMAP-Lite

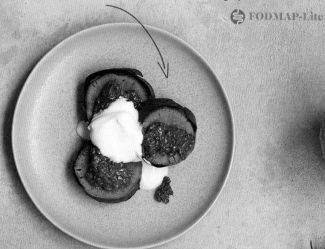

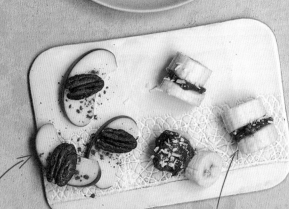

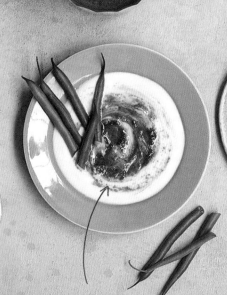

Apple Slider: Apple, pecans, and cinnamon.

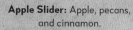 FODMAP-Lite

Banana Bites: Banana slices glued together with nut butter and unsweetened shredded coconut.

FODMAP-Lite

Bean Dippers: Probiotic yogurt with a teaspoon of harissa paste or whole grain mustard stirred through, served with raw green beans or sugar snap peas.

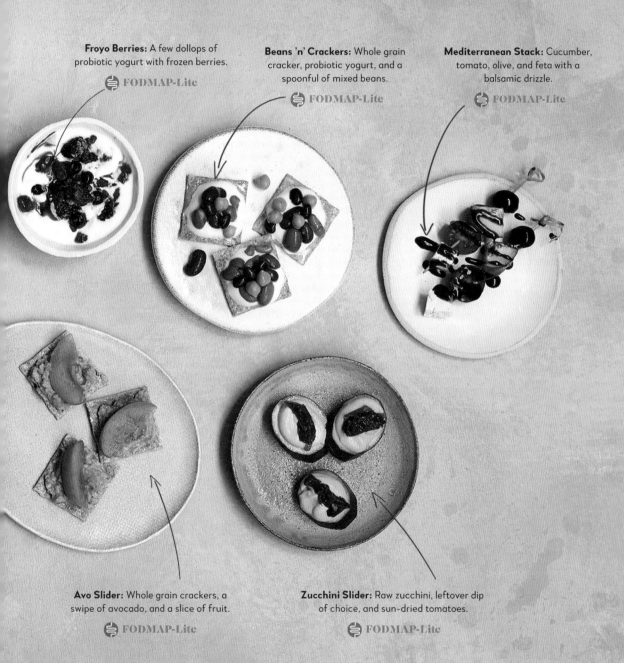

Froyo Berries: A few dollops of probiotic yogurt with frozen berries.

FODMAP-Lite

Beans 'n' Crackers: Whole grain cracker, probiotic yogurt, and a spoonful of mixed beans.

FODMAP-Lite

Mediterranean Stack: Cucumber, tomato, olive, and feta with a balsamic drizzle.

FODMAP-Lite

Avo Slider: Whole grain crackers, a swipe of avocado, and a slice of fruit.

FODMAP-Lite

Zucchini Slider: Raw zucchini, leftover dip of choice, and sun-dried tomatoes.

FODMAP-Lite

FODMAP-Lite Recipe Switches

	Recipe	Portion Size/Switch
Breakfast	Muffin in a Mug (page 140)	Stick to one portion and switch out dates for maple syrup.
	Omelet Bowl (page 141)	Use dried chives instead of onion powder, and use canned peas (rinsed well).
	Fiber-Filled Breakfast Wrap (page 143)	Be sure tofu is firm (not silken); reduce avocado portion to 1 ounce (30 g); switch out whole wheat wrap for gluten-free variety.
	No-Bake Fruit and Nut Bites (page 144)	Stick to a portion of 1 to 2 balls.
	DIY Plant-Packed Granola (page 145)	Opt for rice, corn, or quinoa flakes. Switch out dried mango and apple for dried cranberries or raisins or freeze-dried berries. Stick to a 2-ounce (55 g) portion.
	Crispy Bacon-Shrooms with Creamy Butter Bean Hummus (page 146)	Switch out portobello mushrooms for oyster mushrooms and dates for maple syrup. Spread the hummus thinly; instead of garlic and olive oil, opt for garlic-infused oil. Stick to one slice of sourdough or switch out for a gluten-free option.
	Mango and Berry Froyo Bars (page 148)	Stick to half a portion, and eat with additional probiotic yogurt or FODMAP-lite granola on the side (see DIY Plant-Packed Granola, page 145).
	Plant-Powered Baked Oat Bars (page 150)	Stick to 1 portion. Opt for almond milk, and switch out dates for maple syrup.
	Breakfast Pita Pizza (page 153)	Switch out pita bread for a gluten-free pita/wrap. Use only the green parts of the scallion, and be sure the sun-dried tomatoes don't include garlic or onion. Use half a portion of the base sauce and stick to 1 ounce (30 g) of avocado.
	Eat-the-Rainbow Pancakes (page 155)	Stick to 2 small pancakes, topped with probiotic yogurt and maple syrup.
Sweet Treats	Loaded Melon Wedges (page 159)	Switch out watermelon for honeydew, and stick to 3 ounces (85 g). For the berry whip option: switch out blackberries for blueberries and honey for maple syrup. If using chocolate-hazelnut spread, keep to a 2 tablespoons portion.
	Ultimate Raspberry and White Chocolate Muffins (page 163)	Switch out whole wheat flour for gluten-free flour and dates for maple syrup.

	Recipe	Portion Size/Switch
Light Bites	Garlicky Aquafaba Aioli (page 172)	Switch out garlic for 1 tablespoon of garlic-infused olive oil.
	Smoky Eggplant Dip (page 174)	Switch out garlic and olive oil for garlic-infused olive oil.
	No-Added-Sugar Ketchup (page 175)	Stick to a 2-tablespoon portion and reduce onion to 2 ounces (55 g). Switch out dates for maple syrup.
	Seedy Cracker Duo (page 177)	Switch out rye flour for gluten-free flour.
	Snack-o-Clock Veggie Fritters (page 181)	Switch out whole wheat flour for gluten-free flour, and use vegetable options from page 311.
	All-the-Greens Phyllo Pie (page 182)	Stick to one serving. Use canned peas (rinsed well).
	Popcorn Chick-less Nuggets (page 185)	Switch out whole wheat flour for gluten-free flour.
	Butternut Muffins (page 191)	Switch out spelt flour for gluten-free flour and butternut squash for sweet potato. Stick to a maximum of 3 muffins per portion.
Packed Lunches	Smoked Mackerel, New Potato, and Apple Salad (page 197)	Switch out cashews for nut options (see page 311) and asparagus for green beans. Limit fennel to 6 ounces (170 g), and switch out apples for 7 ounces (200 g) of grapes.
	Baked Sweet Potato with Black Beans (page 198)	Switch out sweet potato for a regular potato and garlic and olive oil for garlic-infused olive oil. Reduce black beans to 3 ounces (80 g) and add 5 ounces (140 g) of chopped tomatoes, peppers, or other veggies (see page 309). Limit avocado to 2 ounces (55 g).
	Baked Sweet Potato with Nut-Free Pesto (page 199)	Switch out sweet potato for regular potato and garlic and olive oil for garlic-infused olive oil. Limit butter beans to 3 ounces (80 g) and add 5 ounces (140 g) of chopped peppers, or other veggies (see page 311).
	PB & J Baked Sweet Potato (page 199)	Stick to half a sweet potato per portion (3 ounces/85 g cooked) and opt for nut or seed butter (see on page 311).

	Recipe	Portion Size/Switch
Packed Lunches	Chunky Veggie and Feta Frittata (page 203)	Replace red onion with the green part of a scallion.
	Tofu Fried Whole Grains with Crunchy Cashews (page 204)	Opt for a gluten-free whole grain (e.g., quinoa, buckwheat, wild rice). Switch out cashews for nuts and stir-fry veggies for other vegetable options (see page 311). Use only the green part of the scallion and canned peas (rinsed well). Switch out silken tofu for firm (or opt for an egg) and garlic for 1 tablespoon of garlic-infused olive oil.
	Reinvented Chicken Burger (page 207)	Use a gluten-free bun.
	Thai-Inspired Fish Cakes and Crunchy Salad (page 212)	Use only the green part of the scallion.
Weeknight Dinners	Stir-Fry Adventures	Protein: If using canned beans, limit to 1.5 ounces (45 g) per serving and add additional firm tofu, peanuts, eggs, fish, or lean meat. Whole grains: Opt for gluten-free whole grains (see page 311). Vegetables: See page 309 for options.
	Indian-Inspired Stir-Fry (page 218)	Switch out garlic and olive oil for garlic-infused olive oil and cauliflower for any suggested veggies on page 311.
	Indonesian-Inspired Stir-Fry (page 219)	Switch out shallots for the green part of a scallion.
	Italian-Inspired Stir-Fry (page 219)	Switch out garlic and olive oil for garlic-infused olive oil.
	Korean-Inspired Stir-Fry (page 220)	Opt for gochujang paste, or go without if sensitive to chile.
	Thai-Inspired Stir-Fry (page 220)	Switch out the garlic and olive oil for garlic-infused olive oil and the sugar snap peas for bok choy or fine green beans. Use only the green part of the scallion.
	Orange-Glazed Roasted Salmon (page 228)	Switch out the garlic for 1½ teaspoons of garlic-infused olive oil, and the date paste for maple syrup. Serve with gluten-free whole grains (see page 311). Use only the green part of the scallion.
	Easy Noodle Soup (page 231)	Use onion- and garlic-free vegetable stock and soba (buckwheat) or rice noodles. Opt for firm tofu rather than silken. Use only the green part of the scallion. Skip the chile if sensitive.

	Recipe	Portion Size/Switch
Fancy Dinners	Spinach and Ricotta Stuffed Shells (page 249)	Stick to half a portion, and switch out the garlic and olive oil for garlic-infused olive oil. Be sure the sun-dried tomatoes and tomato puree don't include onion or garlic. Use gluten-free pasta shells and canned peas (rinsed well).
	Tear-and-Share Bread with Butter Bean Relish (page 250)	Stick to half a portion and use a gluten-free loaf. Switch out the onion for 2 ounces (55 g) of the green part of scallion, and dates for maple syrup.
	Chicken 'n' Veggie Meatballs (page 258)	Use gluten-free bread and only the green part of the scallion.
Sides	Greens and Beans (page 265)	Switch out the garlic and olive oil for garlic-infused olive oil. Reduce beans to just one 15-ounce (425 g) can. Stick to one portion.
	Sticky Parsnips (page 266)	Use only the green part of the scallion. Switch out garlic for 1 tablespoon of garlic-infused olive oil and date paste for maple syrup. Use gluten-free flour.
	Steamed Veggies All-Dressed-Up (page 267)	Only use the avocado pesto. Switch out the garlic and olive oil for garlic-infused olive oil. Opt for gluten-free wraps.
	Spinach Balls with Tahini Sauce (page 270)	Switch out date paste for maple syrup.
	Fried Quinoa with Hoisin Drizzle (page 273)	Switch out the garlic for 1 teaspoon of garlic-infused olive oil and date paste for maple syrup. Use only the green part of the scallions. Skip the chile if sensitive.
Desserts	Raspberry and Lemon Ricotta Cheesecake (page 277)	Switch out the honey for maple syrup.
	Trail Mix Loaf Cake with Yogurt and White Chocolate Glaze (page 278)	Stick to 1 portion. Use gluten-free flour, and switch out the dried mango and figs for cranberries/raisins/goji berries.
	Cream-less Ice Cream, Two Ways (pages 279 to 280)	Hidden veggies: Stick to half a portion, switch out dates for maple syrup, and opt for the chocolate-mint as filling option. No freeze: Stick to 1 portion. Use blueberries, raspberries, or strawberries.
	Prebiotic Rocky Road (page 283)	Stick to 1 portion. Replace the dried mango and figs with 4 ounces (115 g) dried banana chips.
	Pistachio Berry Bursts (page 284)	Stick to 2 or 3 per portion.
	Chocolate Chip Zucchini Cookies (page 291)	Switch out the Medjool dates for maple syrup.

	Recipe	Portion Size/Switch
Drinks	Immunity-Nourishing Smoothie (page 296)	Reduce the orange to 3.5 ounces (100 g) and add 1 teaspoon of maple syrup. Switch out the soy milk for almond milk.
	Frothy Cashew Latte (page 302)	Switch out the cashews for peanuts and the date for maple syrup. If you are sensitive to caffeine, switch to decaf coffee.
One-Minute Snacks	Sweet Potato Slider	Keep to 3 ounces (85 g) of sweet potato, and switch out nut and seed butters (see page 311).
	Prebiotic "Chocolate" Milkshake	Opt for cow's or almond milk, nut and seed butters from page 311, and switch out dates for maple syrup.
	Froyo Berries	Keep to a maximum of 3 ounces (85 g) of berries, and choose between blueberries, cranberries, raspberries, and strawberries.
	Zucchini Slider	Be sure the dip doesn't contain onion or garlic.
	Apple Slider	Switch out apple for 2 ounces (55 g) of banana, honeydew, or fruit options (see page 311).
	Banana Bites	Stick to 2 ounces (55 g) of banana, and opt for nut and seed butters from page 311.
	Avo Slider	Keep to 2 crackers, 1 ounce (30 g) of avocado and 3 ounces (85 g) of fruit options listed on page 309.
	Beans 'n' Crackers	Keep to 2 crackers and 1.5 ounces (45 g) of canned mixed beans (triple-rinsed).

Select Higher-FODMAP Foods to Limit		Examples of Alternatives*
Vegetables	Artichokes, asparagus, broccoli, Brussels sprouts, cabbage, cauliflower, chicory root, garlic, leeks, mushrooms, onions, peas, scallions (white part).	Carrots, chives, cucumber, eggplant, ginger, green beans, kale, peppers, pickled garlic and onion, potatoes, pumpkin, spinach, tomatoes, zucchini.
Fruit	Apples, apricots, blackberries, boysenberries, cherries, dates, figs, mango, nectarines, peaches, pears, persimmons, plums, prunes, watermelon, fruit juice (more than ½ cup/120 ml), foods/drinks with added fruit concentrate.	Blueberries, clementines, grapes, honeydew, kiwi, lemons, limes, oranges, passion fruit, pineapple, raspberries, rhubarb, strawberries. Maximum of 1 piece of any fruit per sitting (equivalent of 3 ounces/85 g fresh, 1 ounce/30 g dried, ½ cup/120 ml juice), with a maximum of three sittings across the day.
Protein sources	Legumes (e.g. baked beans, chickpeas, kidney beans, soy beans), pistachios, and cashews.	All fresh meats (e.g., chicken, fish, lamb), eggs, firm tofu, walnuts, Brazil nuts. Peanuts, sunflower or pumpkin seeds, whole or as nut/seed butters. Canned and (thoroughly) rinsed legumes, contain fewer FODMAPs compared to those boiled from dry. Therefore, small portions (¼ cup per sitting), particularly of canned chickpeas, butter beans, and adzuki beans, are better tolerated. ½ cup of canned lentils is considered low-FODMAP.
Whole grains	Keep to ½ cup of cooked or 1 slice of wheat, barley, or rye-based foods per sitting (including couscous and semolina), with up to three across the day.	Quinoa, rice, buckwheat, millet, oats, polenta.
Other	Agave, honey, high-fructose corn syrup, fructose and low-calorie sweeteners ending in -ol. Added inulin, fructo-oligosaccharide, galacto-oligosaccharide in some yogurts and cereals.	Maple syrup, table sugar (sucrose), glucose.

*This is not a comprehensive list; it's just to give you inspiration. Include all other foods that are not listed on the "higher-FODMAP" column in your diet. Remember that this is a modified version, not the full low-FODMAP diet.

References

Introduction

Evelyn Medawar et al., "The Effects of Plant-Based Diets on the Body and the Brain: A Systematic Review," *Translational Psychiatry* 9, no. 226, September 2019.

The Vegan Society, "Statistics," vegansociety.com.

Chapter 1

Mark L. Heiman and Frank L. Greenway, "A Healthy Gastrointestinal Microbiome Is Dependent on Dietary Diversity," *Molecular Metabolism* 5, no. 5, May 2016, 317—20.

Laura E. Martin, Kristen E. Kay and Ann-Marie Torregrossa, "Bitter-Induced Salivary Proteins Increase Detection Threshold of Quinine, But Not Sucrose," *Chemical Senses* 44, no. 6, July 2019, 379—88.

J. Poore and T. Nemecek, "Reducing Food's Environmental Impacts Through Producers and Consumers," *Science* 360, no. 6392, June 2018, 987—92.

Peter Scarborough et al., "Dietary Greenhouse Gas Emissions of Meat-Eaters, Fish-Eaters, Vegetarians and Vegans in the UK," *Climatic Change* 125, 2014, 179—92.

Walter Willett et al., "Food in the Anthropocene: The EAT-Lancet Commission on Healthy Diets from Sustainable Food Systems," *The Lancet* 393, no. 10170, February 2019, 447—92.

L. A. Wyness et al., "Reducing the Population's Sodium Intake: The UK Food Standard Agency's Salt Reduction Programme," *Public Health Nutrition* 15, no. 2, February 2012, 254—61.

Chapter 2

Francisco Asnicar and Sarah E. Berry, "Microbiome Connections with Host Metabolism and Habitual Diet from 1,098 Deeply Phenotyped Individuals," *Nature Medicine* 27, 2021, 331—32.

Gabriele Berg et al., "Microbiome Definition Re-visited: Old Concepts and New Challenges," *Microbiome* 8, no. 103, 2020.

Jeanelle Boyer and Rui Hai Liu, "Apple Phytochemicals and Their Health Benefits," *Nutrition Journal* 3, no. 5, 2004.

Matteo Briguglio et al., "Dietary Neurotransmitters: A Narrative Review on Current Knowledge," *Nutrients* 10, no. 5, May 2018, 591.

British Nutrition Foundation, "Protein," nutrition.org.uk.

R. Deewatthanawong and C. B. Watkins, "Accumulation of γ-Aminobutyric Acid in Apple, Strawberry and Tomato Fruit in Response to Postharvest Treatments," *Acta Horticulturae* 877, VI International Postharvest Symposium, April 2009.

Emmanuelle Dheilly et al., "Cell Wall Dynamics During Apple Development and Storage Involves Hemicellulose Modifications and Related Expressed Genes," *BMC Plant Biology* 6, no. 201, 2016.

Yan Hou et al., "Anti-Depressant Natural Flavanols Modulate BDNF and Beta Amyloid in Neurons and Hippocampus of Double TgAD Mice," *Neuropharmacology* 58, no. 6, May 2010, 911—20.

Francisco Javier-Ruiz-Ojeda et al., "Effects of Sweeteners on the Gut Microbiota: A Review of Experimental Studies and Clinical Trials," *Advances in Nutrition* 10, suppl. 1, January 2019, S31—48.

Abigail J. Johnson et al., "Daily Sampling Reveals Personalized Diet-Microbiome Associations in Humans," *Cell Host & Microbe* 25, no. 6, June 2019, 789—802.

Mark L. Heiman and Frank L. Greenway, "A Healthy Gastrointestinal Microbiome Is Dependent on Dietary Diversity," *Molecular Metabolism* 5, no. 5, May 2016, 317—20.

V. Juturu, J. P. Bowman and J. Deshpande, "Overall Skin Tone and Skin-Lightening-Improving Effects with Oral Supplementation of Lutein and Zeaxanthin Isomers: A Double-Blind, Placebo-Controlled Clinical Trial," *Clinical, Cosmetic and Investigational Dermatology* 9, 2016, 325—32.

Josephine Kschonsek et al., "Polyphenolic Compounds Analysis of Old and New Apple Cultivars and Contribution of Polyphenolic Profile to the In Vitro Antioxidant Capacity," *Antioxidants* 71, no. 1, January 2018, 20.

François Mariotti and Christopher D. Gardner, "Dietary Protein and Amino Acids in Vegetarian Diets—A Review," *Nutrients*, vol. 11, no. 1, November 2019, p. 2661.

Carlos Augusto Monteiro at al., "Household Availability of Ultra-Processed Foods and Obesity in Nineteen European Countries," *Public Health Nutrition* 21, Special Issue 1: *Ultra Processed Foods*, January 2018, 8—26.

Leonardo Nogueira, "Epicatechin Enhances Fatigue Resistance and Oxidative Capacity in Mouse Muscle," *Journal of Physiology* 589, no. 18, September 2011, 4615—31.

M. Poyet et al., "A Library of Human Gut Bacterial Isolates Paired with Longitudinal Multiomics Data Enables Mechanistic Microbiome Research," *Nature Medicine* 24, September 2019, 1442—52

Marion Salomé et al., "Plant-Protein Diversity Is Critical to Ensuring the Nutritional Adequacy of Diets When Replacing Animal with Plant Protein: Observed and Modeled Diets of French Adults," *Journal of Nutrition* 50, no. 3, March 2020, 536—45.

Ambika Satija et al., "Healthful and Unhealthful Plant-Based Diets and the Risk of Coronary Heart Disease in US Adults," *Journal of the American College of Cardiology* 70, no. 4, July 2017, 411—22.

Bruno Senghor et al., "Gut Microbiota Diversity According to Dietary Habits and Geographical Provenance," *Human Microbiome Journal* 7—8, April 2018, 1—9.

E. Thom, "The Effect of Chlorogenic Acid Enriched Coffee on Glucose Absorption in Healthy Volunteers and Its Effect on Body Mass When Used Long-Term in Overweight and Obese People," *Journal of International Medical Research* 35, no. 6, November 2007, 900—8.

Birgit Wassermann, Henry Muller and Gabriele Berg, "An Apple a Day: Which Bacteria Do We Eat with Organic and Conventional Apples?," *Frontiers in Microbiology*, July 2019.

Anna Wojciechowska et al., "Insitols' Importance in the Improvement of the Endocrine—Metabolic Profile in PCOS," *International Journal of Molecular Sciences* 20, no. 22, November 2019, 5787.

Haixia Zhang et al., "Melatonin in Apples and Juice: Inhibition of Browning and Microorganism Growth in Apple Juice," *Molecules* 23, no. 3, February 2018, 521.

Chapter 3

Lars T. Fadnes et al., "Estimating impact of food choices on life expectancy: A modeling study," *PLoS Medicine*, 2022.

Anne Conolly and Sylvie Craig, *Health Survey for England 2018: Overweight and Obesity in Adults and Children*, NHS Digital, December 2019.

Diabetes UK, "Number of People Living with Diabetes Doubles in Twenty Years," February 2018, diabetes.org.uk.

Food and Agriculture Organization of the United Nations, *The Second Report on the State of the World's Plant Genetic Resources for Food and Agriculture*, 2010, fao.org.

GBD 2017 Diet Collaborators, "Health Effects of Dietary Risks in 195 Countries, 200—2017: A Systematic Analysis for the Global Burden of Disease Study 2017," *The Lancet* 393, no. 10184, May 2019, 1958—72.

Mark L. Heiman and Frank L. Greenway, "A Healthy Gastrointestinal Microbiome Is Dependent on Healthy Diets from Sustainable Food Systems," *The Lancet* 393, no. 17170, February 2019, 447—92.

Susan J. Hewlings and Douglas S. Kalman, "Curcumin: A Review of Its Effects on Human Health," *Foods* 6, no. 10, October 2017, 92.

Jonna Jalanka-Tuovinen et al., "Intestinal Microbiota in Healthy Adults: Temporal Analysis Reveals Individual and Common Core and Relation to Intestinal Symptoms," *PloS One* 6, no. 7, 2011, e23035.

Natasha Khazai, Suzanne E. Judd and Vin Tangpricha, "Calcium and Vitamin D: Skeletal and Extraskeletal Health," *Current Rheumatology Reports* 10, 2008, 110—17.

C. M. Weaver, W. R. Proulx and R. Heaney, "Choices for Achieving Adequate Dietary Calcium with a Vegetarian Diet," *American Journal of Clinical Nutrition* 70, no. 3, September 1999, 543s—48.

Andrew Kingston et al., "Projections of Multi-Morbidity in the Older Population in England to 2035: Estimates from the Population Ageing and Care Simulation (PACSim) Model," *Age and Ageing* 47, no. 3, May 2018, 374—80.

Mental Health Foundation, "Mental Health Statistics: UK and Worldwide," mentalhealth.org.uk.

Ravinder Nagpal et al., "Gut Microbiome and Aging: Physiological and Mechanistic Insights," *Nutrition and Healthy Aging* 4, no. 4, June 2018, 267—85.

S. M. K. Rates, "Plants as Source of Drugs," *Toxicon* 39, no. 5, May 2001, 603—13.

M. Rizwan et al., "Tomato Paste Rich in Lycopene Protects Against Cutaneous Photodamage in Humans in Vivo: A Randomized Controlled Trial," *British Journal of Dermatology* 164, no. 1, January 2011, 154—62.

Jan Philipp Schuchardt and Andreas Hahn, "Intestinal Absorption and Factors Influencing Bioavailability of Magnesium," *Current Nutrition & Food Science* 13, no. 4, 2017, 260—78.

Justin L. Sonnenburg and Erica D. Sonnenburg, "Vulnerability of the Industrialized Microbiota," *Science* 366, no. 6464, October 2019.

Chapter 4

James M. Baker, Layla Al-Nakkash and Melissa M. Herbst-Kralovetz, "Estrogen—Gut Microbiome Axis: Physiological and Clinical Implications," *Maturitas* 103, September 2017, 45—53.

Hui Zhao et al., "Compositional and Functional Features of the Female Premenopausal and Postmenopausal Gut Microbiota," *FEBS Letters* 593, no. 18, July 2019, 2655—64.

Tracey L. K. Bear et al., "The Role of the Gut Microbiota in Dietary Interventions for Depression and Anxiety," *Advances in Nutrition* 11, no. 4, July 2020, 890—907.

Mauro Cozzolino et al., "Therapy with Probiotics and Synbiotics for Polycystic Ovarian Syndrome: A Systematic Review and Meta-Analysis," *European Journal of Nutrition* 59, no. 7, May 2020, 2841—56.

Gabriella d'Ettorre et al., "Challenges in the Management of SARS-CoV-2 Infection: The Role of Oral Bacteriotherapy as Complementary Therapeutic Strategy to Avoid the Progression of COVID-19," *Frontiers in Medicine*, July 2020.

M. C. Flux and Christopher A. Lowry, "Finding Intestinal Fortitude: Integrating the Microbiome into a Holistic View of Depression Mechanism, Treatment, and Resilience," *Neurobiology of Disease* 135, no. 104578, February 2020.

Elizabeth A. Grice and Julia A. Segre, "The Skin Microbiome," *Nature Reviews Microbiology* 9, March 2011, 244—53.

Qiukui Hao, Bi Rong Dong and Taixiang Wu, "Probiotics for Preventing Acute Respiratory Tract Infections," Cochrane Database of Systematic Reviews, February 2015.

Yu He et al., "Main Clinical Features of COVID-19 and Potential Prognostic and Therapeutic Value of the Microbiota in SARS-CoV-2 Infections," *Frontiers in Microbiology*, June 2020.

Felice N. Jacka et al., "A Randomised Controlled Trial of Dietary Improvement for Adults with Major Depression (the "SMILES" trial)," *BMC Medicine* 15, no. 23, January 2017.

Wilhelmina Kalt et al., "Recent Research on the Health Benefits of Blueberries and Their Anthocyanins," *Advances in Nutrition* 11, no. 2, March 2020, 224—36.

Candyce H. Kroenke et al., "Effects of a Dietary Intervention and Weight Change of Vasomotor Symptoms in the Women's Health Initiative," *Menopause: The Journal of the North American Menopause Society* 19, no. 9, September 2012, 980—88.

Derek C. Miketinas et al., "Fiber Intake Predicts Weight Loss and Dietary Adherence in Adults Consuming Calorie-Restricted Diets: The POUNDS Lost (Preventing Overweight Using Novel Dietary Strategies): A Study," *Journal of Nutrition* 149, no. 10, October 2019, 1742—48.

Elena Niccolai et al., "The Gut-brain Axis in the Neuropsychological Disease Model of Obesity: A Classical Movie Revised by the Emerging Director 'Microbiome,'" *Nutrients* 11, no. 1, 2019, 156.

K. Rea, T. G. Dinan and J. F. Cryan, "Gut Microbiota: A Perspective for Psychiatrists," *Neuropsychobiology* 79, no. 1, February 2020, 50—62.

Jason M. Ridlon, "*Clostridium scindens*: A Human Gut Microbe with a High Potential to Convert Glucocorticoids into Androgens," *Journal of Lipid Research* 54, no. 9, September 2013, 2437—49.

Jason Solway et al., "Diet and Dermatology: The Role of a Whole-Food, Plant-Based Diet in Preventing and Reversing Skin Aging," *Journal of Clinical and Aesthetic Dermatology* 13, no. 5, May 2020, 38—43.

Hyun Sun-Yoon et al., "Cocoa Flavanol Supplementation Influences Skin Conditions of Photo-Aged Women: A 24-Week Double-Blind, Randomized, Controlled Trial," *Journal of Nutrition* 146, no. 1, January 2016, 46—50.

Joshua Tarini and Thomas M. S. Wolever, "The Fermentable Fiber Insulin Increases Postprandial Serum Short-Chain Fatty Acids and Reduces Free-Fatty Acids and Ghrelin in Healthy Subjects," *Applied Physiology, Nutrition, and Metabolism*, January 2020.

Christoph A. Thaiss et al., "Persistent Microbiome Alterations Modulate the Rate of Post-Dieting Weight Regain," *Nature* 540, November 2016, 544—51.

Anne Vrieze et al., "Transfer of Intestinal Microbiota from Lean Donors Increases Insulin Sensitivity in Individuals with Metabolic Syndrome," *Gastroenterology* 143, no. 4, October 2012, 913—16.

Benjamin D. Weger et al., "The Mouse Microbiome Is Required for Sex-Specific Diurnal Rhythms of Gene Expression and Metabolism," *Cell Metabolism* 29, no. 2, February 2019, 362—82

Inga Wessels and Lothar Rink, "Micronutrients in Autoimmune Diseases: Possible Therapeutic Benefits of Zinc and Vitamin D," *Journal of Nutritional Biochemistry* 77, no. 108240, March 2020.

Marcus White, "James Lind: The Man Who Helped to Cure Scurvy with Lemons," BBC News, October 2016.

Xuan Zhang et al., "The Gut Microbiota: Emerging Evidence in Autoimmune Diseases," *Trends in Molecular Medicine* 26, no. 9, September 2020, 862—73.

Chapter 5

Neal D. Barnard et al., "A Systematic Review and Meta-Analysis of Changes in Body Weight in Clinical Trials of Vegetarian Diets," *Journal of the Academy of Nutrition and Dietetics* 115, no. 6, June 2015, 954—69.

Sadie B. Barr and Jonathan C. Wright, "Postprandial Energy Expenditure in Whole-Food and Processed-Food Meals: Implications for Daily Energy Expenditure," *Food & Nutrition Research* 54, July 2010.

Julie E. Flood-Obbagy and Barbara J. Rolls, "The Effect of Fruit in Different Forms on Energy Intake and Satiety at a Meal," *Appetite* 52, no. 2, April 2009, 416—22.

Kevin D. Hall et al., "Ultra-Processed Diets Cause Excess Calorie Intake and Weight Gain: An Inpatient Randomized Controlled Trial of *Ad Libitum* Food Intake," *Cell Metabolism* 30, no. 1, July 2019, 67—77.

Miguel A. Martínez-González et al., "A Provegetarian Food Pattern and Reduction in Total Mortality in the PREDIMED Study," *American Journal of Clinical Nutrition* 100, suppl. 1, July 2014, 320S—28.

Janet A. Novotny, Sarah K. Gebauer and David J. Baer, "Discrepancy between the Atwater Factor Predicted and Empirically Measured Energy Values of Almonds in Human Diets," *American Journal of Clinical Nutrition* 96, no. 2, August 2012, 296—301.

Hollie A. Raynor et al., "A Cost-Analysis of Adopting a Healthful Diet in a Family-Based Obesity Treatment Program," *Journal of the Academy of Nutrition and Dietetics* 102, no. 5, May 2002, 645—56.

Chapter 6

Celia Framson et al., "Development and Validation of the Mindful Eating Questionnaire," *Journal of the American Diet Association,* author manuscript, August 2010.

Donna M. Winham et al., "Pinto Bean Consumption Reduces Biomarkers for Heart Disease Risk," *Journal of the American College of Nutrition* 26, no. 3, 2007, 243—49.

Recipes

F. De Alzaa et al., "Evaluation of Chemical and Physical Changes in Different Commercial Oils During Heating," *ACTA Scientific Nutritional Health* 2, no. 6, June 2018.

Elli Callegari et al., "Survival of yogurt bacteria in the human gut," *Applied and Environmental Microbiology* 72, no. 7, July 2006, 5113-17.

Acknowledgments

To The Gut Health Doctor inner community: your heartwarming messages and endless support continue to inspire me every day. Thank you for taking this journey with me.

To Thomas, Claire, and Mom, thank you for your brains, energy and support throughout the whole journey; I couldn't have done it without you. To my little Archie, you really were with me every step of the way, from recipe developing and researching (*in utero*) to photo-shooting and editing; Thank you for sharing Mummy with this book.

To Sofia, Bethan, and Elise, thank you for everything you do for The Gut Health Doctor Community.

To Amy, Hannah, Olivia, Jennifer, Saffron, Carly, The Experiment, Andrew, Katie, and the shoot team: Thank you for sharing your expertise and going that extra mile.

To Jamie and the Jamie Oliver Cookery School: Thank you for being my pandemic heroes and letting us use your space for recipe testing. You saved my gut microbes and me from a lot of stress!

To my research team at King's College London and all the other researchers whose work I've referenced in this book. Your dedication to science and tireless efforts are truly appreciated.

Index

Page numbers in *italics* refer to photos.

About the Author

MEGAN ROSSI, PhD, RD, The Gut Health Doctor, is considered one of the most influential gut health specialists internationally. A practicing dietitian and nutritionist for the last decade with an award-winning PhD in gut health, she is also a leading research fellow at King's College London, where she is currently investigating nutrition-based therapies in gut health, including pre- and probiotics, dietary fibers, plant-based diversity, the low-FODMAP diet and food additives. Megan has been the recipient of several prestigious research awards including from the British Nutrition Foundation, presented by HRH Princess Anne. She is also the founder of The Gut Health Clinic, where she leads a team of gut-specialist dietitians who see clients all over the world, and has created her own gut health food company, Bio&Me, to bridge the gap between science and food industry. She is a two-time instant Sunday Times bestselling author and has also been recognized as Business Insider's Top 100 Coolest People in Food & Drink and named Young Australian Achiever of the Year in the UK 2020.

theguthealthdoctor.com | 🅾 🅵TheGutHealthDoctor | 🅣 TheGutHealthDoc